AROMATHERAPY
WORKBOOK

AROMATHERAPY
WORKBOOK

MARCEL F. LAVABRE

Healing Arts Press
Rochester, Vermont

Healing Arts Press
One Park Street
Rochester, Vermont 05767

Library of Congress Cataloging-in-Publication Data

Lavabre, Marcel.
  Aromatherapy workbook / Marcel Lavabre.
      p.   cm.
  ISBN 0-89281-346-6
  1. Aromatherapy.   I. Title.
  RM666.A68L38   1990
615'.321--dc20   89-19869
                                                                      CIP

Printed and bound in the United States

10 9 8 7 6

Healing Arts Press is a division of Inner Traditions International, Ltd.

Distributed to the book trade in Canada by Book Center, Inc., Montreal, Quebec

Distributed to the health food trade in Canada by Alive Books, Toronto and Vancouver

To my daughter, Melissa.

Contents

Introduction   1

ONE: **Aromatics and Perfumes in History**   **3**
Aromatic Medicine in Egypt   3
Distillation and Alchemy   4
The Renaissance, Decline, and Rebirth   5

TWO: **Aromatherapy: A Multilevel Therapy**   **6**
Scientific Research and Modern Aromatherapy   6
A Holistic Perspective   8
The Aromatics and the Soul   9
Psychotherapy and Aromatherapy: A Wide Open Field   13
Un Je Ne Sais Quoi, Un Presque Rien   14

THREE: **Essential Oils: Extraction, Adulterations**   **16**
Essential Oils in the Plant   16
Traditional Methods of Extraction   17
Adulterations, Problems of Quality   20
Floral Waters, Distillates, Hydrolates   21
Do It Yourself   21
How to Keep Your Essential Oils   22

FOUR: **The Chemistry of Essential Oils**   **23**
The Atomic Saga   23
The Chemistry of Common Essential Oil Constituents   25

FIVE: **How to Use Essential Oils**   **38**
Internal Use   38
External Use   39
Skin Care, Cosmetic Uses   41
Hair Care   44
Aromatic Diffusion, Inhalation   44
Conclusion   47

SIX: **The Essential Oils**   **48**
Synthetics versus Natural: Does It Make Scents?   49
Back to the Botanical Families   51

SEVEN: **Essential Oils in Botanical Families**   **54**

EIGHT: **The Art of Blending**   **97**
The Concept of Synergy   97
The Principles of Blending   98
Doses and Proportions for some Basic Preparations   100
Formulas for Some Common Ailments   103

NINE: **Aromatherapy Reference Tables**   **112**
Essential Oils Reference Table   113
Aromatherapy Therapeutic Index   140

Selected Bibliography   **150**

Resource Guide   **153**

Index of Essential Oils   **157**

Index   **159**

Acknowledgments

To Jean Valnet, one of the main pioneers of aromatherapy who, with his book *The Practice of Aromatherapy*, contributed greatly to the revival of this wonderful art.

To Robert Tisserand, who first spread the word in the English-speaking world.

Special thanks to Henri Viaud, a French distiller from Provence, who was the first to stress the importance of long, low-pressure distillation and the use of pure and natural essential oils from specified botanical origin and chemotypes, and who has not always been credited for his contribution to aromatherapy. Viaud tried to distill practically everything that could be distilled. He was the first to produce a few oils that have recently been introduced on the market (such as St. John's wort and meadowsweet). He also revived the therapeutic use of floral waters. I learned a great deal from this wonderful "honête homme," with his amazing and refreshing curiosity and eagerness for new experiments.

To all the humble producers who provide me with their wonderful oils.

To Jane Kennedy, to Rae Dunphy, to Julia Fischer, and to all my customers, for their trust and continuous support in my enterprise since I moved to the United States in 1981.

To Victoria Edwards and Kurt Schnaubelt, who founded with me the American AromaTherapy Association in 1987.

To all the members of the AATA for their contagious enthusiasm.

To Daniel Penoel for his pioneering works in medical aromatherapy.

To all those involved in the bettering and beautifying of our planetary village.

Introduction

Virtually unknown in the United States only a few years ago, aromatherapy has now become the fastest growing natural healing art in this country. In recent years, this fascinating art has attracted extensive media attention. Aromatherapy is becoming highly fashionable.

But aromatherapy is not just a new trend, a new thing to do, as those who are involved in it can testify.

In Europe, where it began more than 60 years ago, aromatherapy is practiced by medical doctors, nurses, and other health professionals. It is taught to medical students in France and is used by some English nurses in their hospitals. Extensive clinical research is underway, mainly in these two countries.

When people first hear about aromatherapy they think about fragrance, perfumes, an alluring world of imagination, magic, fantasy. Quite simply, aromatherapy consists of using essential oils for healing.

Essential oils are volatile oily substances; they are highly concentrated vegetal extracts that contain hormones, vitamins, antibiotics, and antiseptics. In a way, essential oils represent the spirit, the soul of the plant. They are the most concentrated form of herbal energy. Many plants produce essential oils. They are contained in tiny droplets between the cells and play an important role in the biochemistry of the plants. They are also responsible for the fragrance of the plants.

Essential oils are used in cosmetics and pharmacy as well as in perfumery. Their field of activity is quite wide: from deep therapeutic action to the extreme subtlety of genuine perfumes.

In aromatherapy, the essential oils can be taken internally in their pure form or diluted in alcohol, mixed with honey, or in medical preparations. They are used externally in frictions (localized massage), massage, and inhalations. Finally, they are ingredients of numerous cosmetics and perfumes.

Essential oils can have strictly allopathic effects (meaning that they act like regular medicines); more subtle effects, like those of Bach flower remedies or homeopathic preparations; and psychological and spiritual effects, which constitute their most traditional use. They also are powerful antiseptics and antibiotics that are not dangerous for the body. Aromatherapy is thus, in many cases, an excellent alternative to more aggressive therapies.

Essential oils are the "quintessences" of the alchemists. In this sense, they condense the spiritual and vital forces of the plants in a material form. Therefore, they act on the biological level to strengthen the natural defenses of the body and are the media of a direct human-plant communication on the energetic and spiritual plane.

Aromatherapy can be used at many different levels. Essential oils are extremely versatile materials: they are both medicine and fragrance; they can cure the most severe physical condition; they can reach to the depth of our souls.

Before you start reading this book, though, I should warn you: Once you step into the world of essences, you will be exposed to one of the most delightful and harmless forms of addiction. Chances are that you will want to know more and more about this amazing healing art. If you allow yourself to be touched by the power of these wonderful substances, you will discover a new world that is actually very old—the almost forgotten world of nature's fragrances. This is a world without words, a world of images, that you explore from the tip of your nose to the center of your brain—a world of subtle surprises and silent ecstasy.

ONE

Aromatics and Perfumes in History

Since the earliest ages of humanity, aromatic fumigations have been used in daily rituals and during religious ceremonies as an expression and a reminder of an all-pervasive sacredness. Fragrance has been seen as a manifestation of divinity on the earth, a connection between human beings and the gods, medium and mediator, emanation of matter and manifestation of spirit.

AROMATIC MEDICINE IN EGYPT

Aromatic medicine itself emerged from the shade of smoky temples in Egypt—the birthplace of medicine, perfumery, and pharmacy—more than six thousand years ago. The precious substances came from all parts of the world, carried by caravans or by boats: cedar from Lebanon; roses from Syria; spikenard, myrrh, frankincense, labdanum, and cinnamon from Babylon, Ethiopia, Somalia, and even Persia and India.

The priest supervised the preparations in the temples, reading the formulas and chanting incantations while the students mixed the ingredients. Pulverization, maceration, and other operations could continue for months until the right subtle fragrance was obtained for ceremonial use.

But spiritual matters were not the only concern of the Egyptians. They attached the greatest importance to health and hygiene and were thoroughly familiar with the effects of perfumes and aromatic substances on the body and the psyche. Many preparations were used for both their fragrant quality and their healing power. Kephi, for example, a perfume of universal fame, was an antiseptic, a balsamic, and a tranquilizer that could be taken internally.

The Egyptians also practiced the art of massage and were famous specialists in skin care and cosmetology. Their products were renowned all over the civilized world.

The Phoenician merchants exported rich

unguents, scented oils, creams, and aromatic wines all over the Mediterranean world and the Arabic peninsula and thereby enhanced the fame and wealth of Egypt.

Embalming was one of the main uses of aromatics. Bodies were filled with perfumes, resins, and fragrant preparations after removal of the internal organs. So strong is the antiseptic power of essential oils that the tissues are still well preserved thousands of years later. In the seventeenth century, mummies were sold in Europe, and doctors distilled them and used them as ingredients in numerous medicines.

The use of aromatics spread from Egypt to Israel, Greece, Rome, and the whole Mediterranean world. Every culture and civilization, from the most primitive to the most sophisticated, developed its own practice of perfumery and cosmetics. India is probably the only place in the world where the tradition was never lost. With over 10,000 years of continuous practice, Ayurvedic medicine is the oldest continuous form of medical practice.

The Vedas, the most sacred book of India and one of the oldest known books, mention over 700 different products, such as cinnamon, spikenard, coriander, ginger, myrrh, and sandalwood. The Vedas codify the uses of perfumes and aromatics for liturgical and therapeutic purposes.

DISTILLATION AND ALCHEMY

In Europe, the advent of Christianity and the fall of the Roman Empire marked the beginning of a long period of barbarism and a general decline of all knowledge. Revival came from the Arabic countries with the advent of Islam. Intellectual and cultural activity flourished, as did the arts. Arabic civilization attained an unequaled degree of refinement.

The philosophers devoted themselves to the old hermetic art of alchemy, whose origin was attributed to the Egyptian god Tehuti. They revived the use of aromatics in medicine and perfumery and perfected the techniques. The great philosopher Avicenna invented the refrigerated coil, a real breakthrough in the art of distillation.

Alchemy, which was probably introduced to Europe by the crusaders on their way back from the Holy Land, was primarily a spiritual quest, and the different operations performed by the adept were symbolic of the processes taking place within himself. Distillation was the symbol of purification and the concentration of spiritual forces.

In the alchemist's vision, everything, from sand and stones to plants and people, was made up of a physical body, a soul, and spirit. In accordance with the basic principle "solve and coagula" (dissolve and coagulate), the art of "spagyrie" consisted of dissolving the physical body and condensing the soul and spirit, which had all the curative power, into the quintessences. The material was distilled over and over to remove all impurities, and the final products were highly potent medicines.

With the expansion of this mysterious art, more and more substances were treated for the extraction of essences. These quintessences were the basis of most medicines, and for centuries essential oils remained the only remedies for epidemic diseases.

THE RENAISSANCE, DECLINE, AND REBIRTH

During the Renaissance, the use of essential oils expanded into perfumery and cosmetics. With further progress in the arts of chemistry and distillation, the production of elixirs, balms, scented waters, fragrant oils, and unguents for medicine and skin care flourished. Nicholas Lemery, the personal physician of Louis XIV, described many such preparations in his *Dictionnaire des Drogues Simples*. Some have survived until now: Melissa water, Arquebuse water, and the famous Cologne water, for instance, are still produced.

The advent of modern science in the nineteenth century marked the decline of all forms of herbal therapy. The early scientists had a simplistic and somewhat naive vision of the world. When the first alkaloids were discovered, scientists thought it better to keep only the main active principles of the plants, to reproduce them in laboratories. Thus they discovered and reproduced penicillin (from a natural mold growing on bread), aspirin (naturally present in birch, wintergreen, and meadowsweet), antibiotics, and so on.

Without denying the obvious value of many scientific discoveries, we must acknowledge that the narrow vision of the medical profession has led to some abuses. Microorganisms adapt much faster to antibiotics than does the human body, making antibiotics inefficient as well as dangerous to the body. Corticosteroids have dreadful side effects; hypnotics, antidepressants, and amphetamines are highly addictive; and so on.

At the beginning of this century, a few convinced explorers started to investigate with the scientific tools the old knowledge accumulated through the ages—knowledge that had been scornfully dismissed. R. M. Gattefosse founded aromatherapy, followed by Dr. M. Fesneau, Professor Caujolles, and Dr. Pellecuer, to name a few.

The expansion of aromatherapy in Europe really started in 1964 with the publication of Dr. Jean Valnet's book *Aromatherapie* (translated as *The Art of Aromatherapy*, Healing Arts Press, Rochester, Vermont, 1982). Today, aromatherapy is a very active movement in France, with practitioners such as Professor Pradal, Dr. Girault, and Dr. Belaiche in the medical circles, and Dr. Lamblin, Professor Lautie, P. Passebeck, and P. Franchomme in the naturopathic movement. Aromatherapy is practiced by medical doctors, and essential oils can be found in any health food store and most pharmacies. Their purchase is reimbursed by French health insurance.

TWO

Aromatherapy:
A Multi-Level Therapy

SCIENTIFIC RESEARCH AND MODERN AROMATHERAPY

Modern aromatherapy was born at the turn of the century from the works of the French chemist R. M. Gattefosse and has since attracted interest in France, Germany, Switzerland, and Italy. Many studies have been made by laboratory scientists and by practicing therapists. Most of this research, somewhat constrained by the dominant scientific ideology, almost exclusively concerns the antiseptic and antibiotic powers of essential oils and their allopathic properties.

Since the early 1980s, however, with the work of Dr. Schwartz at Yale University, and of professors Dodd and Van Toller at Warwick University in England, a better understanding of the mechanisms of olfaction has opened new, exciting avenues for research and experimentation in aromatherapy.

The Antiseptic Power of Essential Oils

After Pasteur, belief in external agents (microbes, spores, viruses) as the cause of diseases became the basic assumption of official medicine. It was natural, in this context, that the first studies of essential oils should concern their antiseptic properties. Koch himself studied the action of turpentine on *Bacillus anthracis* in 1881; in 1887 Chamberland studied the action of the essential oils of oregano, cinnamon, and clove buds. Other studies by Rideal and Walker, and Kellner and Kober, proposed different methods of measuring the antiseptic power of essential oils in direct contact or in their vaporized states.

The Aromatogram

With the aromatogram, Dr. Maurice Girault

went one step further and provided a useful tool for prescription and diagnosis. Girault, a French gynecologist and obstetrician, has studied the effects of essential oils and tinctures (in association with other natural therapies – homeopathy, minerals, etc.) in gynecology for 20 years. The results of his work were published in *Traite de Phytotherapie et d'Aromatherapie*, vol. 3, *Gynecologie*, Maloine Editeur, Paris, 1979.

In the aromatogram, vaginal secretions on a swab are tested against several essential oils to determine which oil is the most efficient against the specific microorganism. This method has been extended to all infectious disease by French aromatherapy doctors Pradal, Belaiche, Andoui, and Durrafour. It has the advantage of dealing with real germs coming from real sites in real patients, rather than from laboratories.

Virtually No Resistance Phenomena

For all their imperfections and limitations, the various methods of analyzing the germicidal power of essential oils have given scientific validation to aromatherapy. The action of essences on microorganisms is now better understood: essences inhibit certain metabolic functions of microorganisms, such as growth and multiplication, eventually destroying them if the inhibition continues.

Even though there is general agreement on the antiseptic power of essential oils, different authors classify them differently by their antigenetic properties. Since essential oils are products of life, their chemical composition depends on so many factors that it is impossible to get exactly the same essence twice. Therefore, different analyses will give different results. According to Jean Valnet, microorganisms show no resistance to essential oils. Recent research on the subject suggests that there are resistance phenomena; but to a far lesser degree than to synthetic antibiotics. This makes sense, as essential oils have a more complex structure and moreover are produced by the defense mechanisms of the plant.

The Power of Living Substances

The real interest of essential oils in medicine lies in their action on the site. If they could easily and advantageously be replaced by synthetic products for their antiseptic uses, these synthetics would always be awkward in their interaction with the body as a whole, even though synthetics are chemical reconstructions of components naturally occurring in essential oils.

Essential oils have hundreds of chemical components, most of them in very small amounts. We know that certain trace elements are fundamental for life. In the same way, the power of living products lies in the combination of their elements, and their trace components are at least as important as their main components. No synthetic reconstruction can fully replicate a natural product. It is thus very important to always use natural essential oils.

A HOLISTIC PERSPECTIVE

The human body is a whole, and the interactions taking place between the whole, its parts, and the environment are regulated according to a principle of equilibrium called homeostasis.

Homeostasis is an autoregulation process that is ensured by such substances as hormones, and the secretions of endocrine glands controlled by the corticohypothalamo-hypophyseal complex. Any external or internal aggression brings a compensatory regulation (hyper- or hypo-functioning) and an imbalance that provokes a defense reaction. The ingestion of chemicals is often an aggression. In disease, chemotherapy consists in answering one aggression with another, creating a state of war highly prejudicial to the battleground—the human body!

We depend on plants in every domain—food, energy, and oxygen—and there is between plants and humans a complementary relationship. We are part of the same whole, which is life itself. This is why plants are not aggressive to the body. (Only their abuse can be aggressive.)

Hippocrates, the father of occidental medicine, founded his practice on two basic principles: the principle of similarities (treat the same with the same, the poison with the poison), and the principle of oppositions (find antidotes). The latter, quite straightforward in its application, is the basis of modern medicine (allopathy). The former requires intuition and subtlety; it inspired the theory of similarities as formulated by the great alchemist and philosopher Paracelsus in the Middle Ages. It is also the basic principle of homeopathy and anthroposophic medicine.

From observing the morphology of plants and their different characteristics (smell, taste, area where they grow, environment, soil, overall vibration), Paracelsus could predict their therapeutic indications. Rudolph Steiner and the anthroposophists adopted the same methods. Their findings have been amazingly accurate and have been largely confirmed by scientific research.

Theories of information and genetics, dealing with the issues of order and chaos, give further justification to such an approach. According to these theories, adaptability and mobility in the use of information are among the chief characteristics of life. A living system (a cell, an organism, a colony of insects, a social group) starts with a certain range of potentials that become actual in a feedback process with the environment. Thus, the embryo and the human being develop from a single primordial cell by differentiation. Life, on the other hand, apparently uses universal structures (such as chromosomic or enzymatic structures). Living systems seem able to "borrow" information from other living systems; to some extent, they are able to incorporate alien information.

If the clue to recovery lies within oneself, it should be very beneficial to give the right kind of information to the body. Therefore, close investigation of the role of essential oils in plants will help one understand their curative power, while the observation of specific plants will tell us about the healing properties of each individual oil.

Essential oils evidently play a key role in the biochemistry of the plant; they are like hormones contained in small "bags" located between the cells, and they act as regulators and messengers. They catalyze biochemical reactions, they protect the plant from parasites and diseases, and they play an important role in fertilization. (Orchids, the most fascinating family of plants, have developed the process to a high degree, attracting the most suitable insects to carry precious pollen to their remote sexual partners.)

Essential oils carry information between the cells and are related to the hormonal response of the plant to stressful situations. They are agents of the plant's adaptation to its environment. It is not surprising, then, that they contain hormones. Sage, traditionally known to regulate and promote menstruation, contains estrogen. Ginseng, a well-known tonic and aphrodisiac, contains substances similar to estrone. Estrogens can also be found in parsley, hops, and licorice. Rosemary increases the secretion of bile and facilitates its excretion.

Essential oils control the multiplication and renewal of cells. They have cytophilactic and healing effects on the human body (especially lavender, geranium, garlic, hyssop, and sage). According to Jean Valnet, they have anticarcinogenic properties.

They are often present in the outer part of leaves, in the skin of citrus fruits, and in the bark of certain trees. Cosmetic applications are among their oldest uses.

Most aromatic plants grow in dry areas, and the essential oils in them are produced by solar activity. In the anthroposophic vision, essential oils are the manifestation of the fire cosmic forces. They are produced by the plant's cosmic self. In them, matter dissolves into warmth. Therefore, they are indicated for diseases originating in the astral body.

THE AROMATICS AND THE SOUL

Aromatherapy acts at different levels. There is first an allopathic action due to the chemical composition of the essential oils and their antiseptic, stimulant, calming, antineuralgic, or other properties. There is a more subtle action at the level of information, similar to the action of homeopathic or anthroposophic remedies. Last but not least, essential oils act on the mind. In fact, they are most traditionally used as basic ingredients of perfumes. Generally speaking, pleasant odors have obvious uplifting effects. According to Marguerite Maury in *The Secret of Life and Youth*:

> Of the greatest interest is the effect of fragrances on the psychic and mental state of the individual. Power of perception becomes clearer and more acute, and there is a feeling of having, to a certain extent, outstripped events. . . .It might even be said that the emo-

tional trouble which in general obscures our perception is practically suppressed.

Anatomy of Olfaction

Recent research conducted in Europe, the United States, and the Soviet Union reveals that the effects of odors on the psyche may be more important than scientists have suspected. The University of Warwick, England, has been conducting fascinating research on this subject (see Theimer, *Fragrance Chemistry: The Science of the Sense of Smell*). Figure 1 illustrates the anatomy of olfaction.

The sense of smell acts mostly on a subconscious level; the olfactory nerves are directly connected to the most primitive part of the brain, the limbic system—our connection with our remote saurian ancestors, our distant reptile cousins. In a sense, the olfactory nerve is an extension of the brain itself, which can then be reached directly through the nose. This is the only such open gate to the brain.

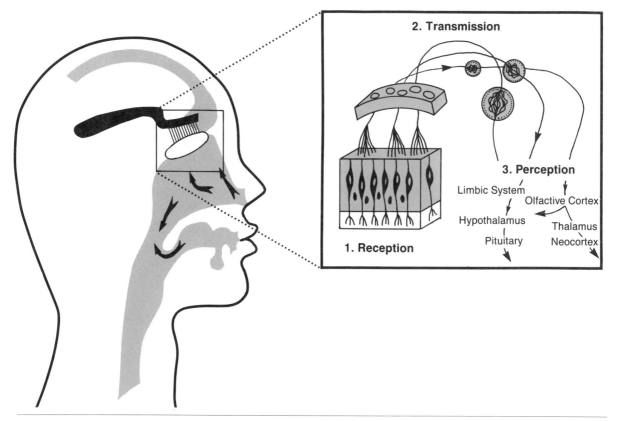

Fig. 1 The Anatomy of Olfaction

The limbic system, originally known as the rhinencephalon ("smell brain"), is the part of the brain that regulates the sensoimotor activity and deals with the primitive drives of sex, hunger, and thirst. Stimulation of the olfactory bulb sends electrical signals to the area of the limbic system concerned with visceral and behavioral mechanisms; they directly affect the digestive and sexual systems and emotional behavior. In fact, the brain's electrical response to odors is about the same as the one correlated with emotions. (In the French language the same verb, *sentir*, is used for "to smell" and "to feel.") The processes of olfactory reception are largely unconscious; we are mostly unaware of our scentual environment. For some yet unexplained reason, whenever we are in contact with a new odor, we become "blind" to it after a while. The electrical signals correlated to this odor still continue to reach the brain, but the contacts with our conscious centers have been shut off. This shows how little control our conscious centers have on the olfactory stimulations.

The sense of smell is very sensitive: we can detect up to one part of fragrant material in 10,000 billion parts or more. A trained nose can differentiate several hundred different odors. However, we have no proper vocabulary to talk about odors. We say that something smells like rose, strawberry, skunk, or whatever. The olfactory nerves terminate in a part of the brain that does not use the same kind of logic as our intellectual centers. Although odors form a kind of communication system, they cannot be developed as a language; they work through associations and images and are not analytical.

In *Perfumery: The Psychology and Biology of Fragrances*, E. Douek describes various olfactory abnormalities. According to the author, anosmia, the total inability to smell, is always accompanied by some elements of depression, which can often become severe. With loss of the sense of smell, people also lose the sense of taste. The world becomes dull and colorless.

Even more interesting is parosmia, or olfactory illusion (usually related to a perception of bad odors). In such cases, shy and withdrawn people tend to feel that the unpleasant odors they perceive emanate from themselves, while people with paranoid tendencies perceive them as coming from others. The latter suspect imaginary plots in their associates and generally show tyrannical tendencies. According to Douek, the French king Louis XI suffered from this affliction. He was very good at filling up his prisons and inventing sophisticated tortures to obtain confessions from his victims. It might well be instructive to investigate the olfactory sanity of the most prominent tyrants throughout history!

Olfactory System and Sexual Mechanisms

Mammals release sexual olfactory signals called pheromones through specialized scent-producing apocrine glands. In humans, most of these glands are located in the circumanal and anogenital region, the chest and the abdomen, and around the nipples, with some variations between the different races. (According to D. M. Stoddart, pheromone production is minimal among Mongoloids, especially Korean Huanghoids.)

D. M. Stoddart notes that most perfumes contain ingredients that mimic these sexual olfactory signals, such as civet, musk, or castoreum, and also substances like sandalwood (remarkably similar, according to the author, to androsterol, a male human pheromone). According to G. H. Dodd, humans secrete musk-like molecules, and therefore we experience this type of odor in utero, which could explain the universal liking for it. The main function of perfumes would then be to heighten and fortify natural odors, rather than to cover them.

The connection between olfaction and the sexual system takes place through the hypothalamic region. According to D. M. Stoddart in *Perfumery: The Psychology and Biology of Fragrance*:

> The hypothalamic region is a major receiver of olfactory neurones, and releases a variety of . . . hormones which pass to the anterior pituitary via the hypophyseal portal system, and induces the pituitary to secrete the suite of hormones which governs and controls the mammalian sexual cycles.

The synchronization of menstrual periods in girl's boarding schools is a well-known phenomenon. Several studies have shown that such synchronicity could be caused by axillary secretions (i.e., by pheromones).

In another now famous experiment, set up in a kindergarten, children playing near a pile of T-shirts worn by their mothers could accurately find their own mother's T-shirts within a very short time. Most of them would then retire to a corner with the T-shirt and quiet down. Although this experiment is not directly concerned with sexual matters, it shows the strong olfactory component of the mother-infant bond. It is also worth noting that breast-fed babies develop a much stronger olfactory bond to their mother than do bottle-fed ones.

The Gate to the Soul

When Sigmund Freud opened the Pandora's box of the unconscious at the beginning of this century, he suspected sexual drives to be the central feature of the show being played on our private stage. He considered the repression of smell to be a major cause of mental illness and suspected that the nose was related to the sexual organs. (Allergy to odors is a psychosomatic disease.)

If psychoanalysis and its avatars are to explore the unconscious from the mental side, the nose and the sense of smell give access to Pandora's box from the other side: the unknown side, the saurian side, from the origin of ages. The subtle emanations create a diffuse network that connects us to the unconscious of species, and to life itself. The strongest and deepest experiences are often accompanied by olfactory sensations. All traditions, even the most puritan, have known the power of fragrances; every religion knew their ceremonial use (usually in connection with sounds and colors) to generate elation among the faithful. The holy man, the mystic, experiences heavenly fragrances in his deepest ecstasy. Such people may eventually die in the "odor of sanctity."

Fragrances can bring about the deepest but most fugitive sensations. Like happiness, or love, or laughter, they catch you, almost by surprise, and fade away as soon as you try to grasp them. As you walk along the street, pull out the weeds in your backyard, hike on a trail, or sip your coffee, a mysterious emanation suddenly strikes your nose and the magic unfolds. In an instant of rapture, waves of delight run through your entire body, bringing about images and new sensations. But if you try to figure out what is going on, the experience disappears like a soap bubble; if you try to talk about it, you will soon fall short of words.

According to Jean-Jacques Rousseau, the sense of smell is imagination itself. Some authors needed olfactory sensations to stimulate their creativity. Guy de Maupassant, for instance, used to soak strawberries in a bowl of ether. Schiller filled the top drawer of his desk with ripe apples.

The sense of smell is closely related to memory; olfactory memories are very accurate and almost indelible. A French psychoanalyst, Andre Virel, used fragrance to bring forth hidden memories. The odor and taste of a madeleine dipped in a cup of tea inspired Marcel Proust to write one of the most remarkably precise and vivid works of introspection, and a masterpiece of literature.

We probably all have our own private madeleines. Syringa, to me, is one of the most heavenly fragrances. It transports me to a space of undisturbed peacefulness where I can vividly recall the vegetable garden of my early childhood, with its fallen trellis, its dry wall above the dirt road leading to the spring, and its basin of fresh running water. There is a huge fig tree in the corner just above the road and stone shed, falling in ruins on the other side with a bush of syringa in the middle. I am leaning against the bush now in full bloom; I have been here for hours. Out there, behind the stone arch, is the farm, and then the world. But here, the warm and gentle sun of May envelops my frail body; the divine fragrance of syringa bathes my soul. I am at totally home. Why should I ever move?

PSYCHOTHERAPY AND AROMATHERAPY: A WIDE OPEN FIELD

Since the olfactory system is such an open gate to the subconscious, one would expect that psychotherapy could benefit from the use of olfactory stimuli for the cure of psychological disorders. Very little research has been done in this area, however, possibly because it is hard to systematize any kind of therapeutic procedure. The sense of smell is very private. Each individual's associations are different. Dr. A. D. Armond, for instance reported the case of an anxious patient who worked on motor bikes and kept an oily washer in his pocket for comfort in times of stress. Still, aromatherapy can offer some valuable tools to the practitioner. Oils such as neroli, lavender, marjaram, rose, and ylang ylang have been traditionally used for their calming effects in stress reduction. Jasmine is a wonderful uplifting oil for the treatment of depression or anxiety, and there are many more (see the study of the individual oils and the therapeutic index). Diffusion is probably one of the best methods of using essential oils in this way.

One procedure often used by therapists is to prepare an appropriate blend of oils to use during the therapeutic session. The patient can then use the same blend at home to further the treatment. This method is particularly efficient when used in conjunction with any technique conducive to deep relaxation (such as hypnosis, meditation, yoga, or certain types of massage), as the olfactory stimuli are then more likely to have a deep impact on the patient.

Obviously, psychoaromatherapy (a term coined by Robert Tisserand) is still a wide-open field, where experimentation should be encouraged. With minimal caution, no adverse side effects can be expected from the use of aroma in psychotherapy, while the potential benefits appear to be unlimited. I am personally very curious about any finding in this fascinating domain and invite my therapist readers to share their experience in this area with me or with the American AromaTherapy Association (see resource guide).

UN JE NE SAIS QUOI, UN PRESQUE RIEN

Essential oils and fragrances have been extensively used for well-being—one of the main keys to health—since the beginning of civilization.

Vladimir Jankelevitch, a French philosopher who used to give cooking classes to his delighted students in the venerable Sorbonne, talked about *un je ne sais quoi, un presque rien* ("an I-don't-know-what, an almost-nothing") to characterize the subtle quality of an *art de vivre*, which can be extended to the basic jubilation of just being alive. This *je ne sais quoi*, this *presque rien* that is the mark of genuine art, of elegance, of humor, which differentiates a real meal from a mere quantity of proteins, calories, vitamins, and minerals, describes perfectly the contribution of fragrances to the quality of life. It is unpredictable, it cannot be analyzed by any scientific method, and yet it can be experienced. According to Goethe, the most evolved plants go through a transformation from the primitive germ to the exuberance of the flower in a natural movement toward spirituality where the flower, in its impermanence and openness, represents an instant of rapture and jubilation. Fragrance is a manifestation of this jubilation.

Fragrances have their own language.

Better than any word, they can express the most subtle feelings. Much is revealed about a person by his or her choice of fragrance and how that fragrance reacts with the skin. Everyone has his or her specific odor, which changes depending on the physical and mental state of the individual. Thus, dogs can find lost people and criminals. Smell may, in fact, be a determinant in the establishment of relationships. It has also been a traditional tool for diagnosis (each disease is said to have its specific odor).

Aromas, even if they cannot change an individual, may help to create a favorable ground if properly chosen. Fragrances stimulate the dynamic and positive aspect of the being by an effect of resonance. During the Renaissance, the *grande dames* had their own secret perfumes; numerous systems associate perfumes with astrological signs, dominant planets, or morphological characteristics.

In conclusion, even though it can relieve symptoms, aromatherapy primarily aims at curing the causes of diseases. The main therapeutic action of essential oils consists in strengthening the organs and their functions, and acting on the defense mechanisms of the body. They do not do the job for the body; they help the body do its own job and thus do not weaken the organism. Their action is enhanced by all natural therapies that aim to restore the vitality of the individual. Maurice Girault recommended using them in connection with minerals, homeopathy, and psychotherapy. I would definitely add nutrition, as food is the basis of animal life; depending on its quality, food can be the best medicine or the main cause of disease.

THREE

Essential Oils:
Extraction, Adulterations

ESSENTIAL OILS IN THE PLANT

Essential oils are more or less fluid (some of them are solid at room temperature). They differ from fatty oils in being highly volatile. Thus, if you put a drop of essential oil on a piece of cloth or paper, the stain disappears after a while (between a few minutes and a few days). The oils are often colored and are usually lighter than water. They do not dissolve in water and are slightly soluble in vinegar. They dissolve fairly well in alcohol and mix very well with vegetable oils, fats, and waxes. Essential oils are contained in many plants; they are especially abundant in Labiatae, Myrtaceae, Coniferae, Rutaceae, Lauraceae, and Umbelliferae. They are present in tiny droplets between the cells, where they act as hormones, regulators, and catalysts. They appear to aid the plant in adapting to its environment and thus increase their yield in situations that are stressful to the plant.

In extreme climates, such as the Arabian desert, certain plants use essential oils as a protection against the sun. Myrrh and frankincense bushes are surrounded by a very thin cloud of essential oils, which filters the sun's rays and freshens the air around the bushes. *Dictamus fraxinella*, a plant of the same family that grows in the Sinai, is so liberally endowed with resinous oil glands that the resinous vapor perpetually surrounding the shrub burns with a brilliant glow when lit. (According to Roy Genders, the burning bush that Moses saw in the Sinai could have been caused by such a phenomenon.) Essential oils protect the plant from diseases and parasites. They attract certain insects for pollination. They sometimes even act as natural selective weedkillers, creating a territory around their roots where certain other plants cannot grow. Organic and biodynamic farmers know how to take advantage of this phenomenon in their work: certain plants have dynamic effects on the growth of specific plants while inhibiting others.

The chemistry of essential oils is rather complex. It varies during the day and throughout the year; it depends on the part of the plant being distilled (root, wood, bark, leaf, stem, flower, seed), the variety, the soil, even the climate. The oils are mainly constituted of terpenes, sesquiterpenes, esters, alcohols, phenols, aldehydes, ketones, and organic acids. They contain vitamins, hormones, antibiotics, and/or antiseptics. The yield of essential oils varies between 0.005% and 10% of the plant. Thus, one pound of essential oil requires 50 pounds of eucalyptus or lavandin, 150 pounds of lavender, 500 pounds of sage, thyme, or rosemary, and 2000 to 3000 pounds of rose!

TRADITIONAL METHODS OF EXTRACTION

Enfleurage

Extraction by fats is probably the oldest method of obtaining essential oils. Cold extraction consists in soaking the plants in vegetable oil in a glass jar and exposing them to the sun for 1 or 2 weeks. The plants are then strained out, and more herbs are added to the scented oil. Shepherds and farmers in Provence, in southeast France, prepare the "red oil" by soaking St. John's wort flowers in olive oil for 2 weeks. This oil has amazing healing properties and is very efficient against burns.

In enfleurage, another method of extraction, a layer of fresh flowers is placed on an oil-soaked cloth or a thin layer of lard. The flowers are replaced by fresh ones every day until the right concentration is obtained.

Though these different methods do not allow a separation of the essential oils, the products obtained are particularly suited to creams, ointments, liniments, massage oils, bath oils, etc.

Cold Expression

Some essential oils can be extracted by cold pressure; this process is commonly used for citrus fruits. (If you pinch the peel of a lemon or an orange in front of a candle flame, you can see the oil come out when it burns in the flame.)

The Origin of Distillation

Distillation is still the most common process of extracting essential oils. Historians do not agree on its origin, but most attribute it to Avicenna, the famous Arab philosopher, physician, and alchemist, who lived at the turn of the millennium. However, Zozime, renowned Egyptian chemist living in the third century A.D., wrote about numerous designs of stills adorning the wall of a temple in Memphis. It is quite likely, in fact, that the Egyptians were aware of a primitive process of distillation.

In the first century A.D., Dioscorides already wondered about the origin of distillation. He reported that according to oral tradition, a physician baked pears between two dishes. When he took off the upper dish, he noticed that the steam covering it smelled and tasted like a pear. It inspired him to build elaborate instruments for the extraction of the "quintessences" of medicinal plants.

A still consists of a vat: a large cylindrical tank, which contains the plants. Steam is sent through the plants from the bottom of the vat and evaporates the oils. The vat is covered by a special lid (*col de cygne* or swan neck), which collects the steam and sends it to the coil, usually refrigerated with

running water, where the steam is condensed. The mixture of condensed water and oil separates naturally by decantation in *vase florentin* (florentine vase). This is illustrated in Figure 2.

Many farms in southeastern France had such equipment until the turn of the century. Relatively small (the main vat contained less than 100 gallons), they were often used for extracting essential oils (mostly wild lavender) in the summer and distilling brandy in the winter. Today, wild lavender has almost disappeared and nobody picks it any more (I bought one of the last batches a few years ago), but there are still many distiller-

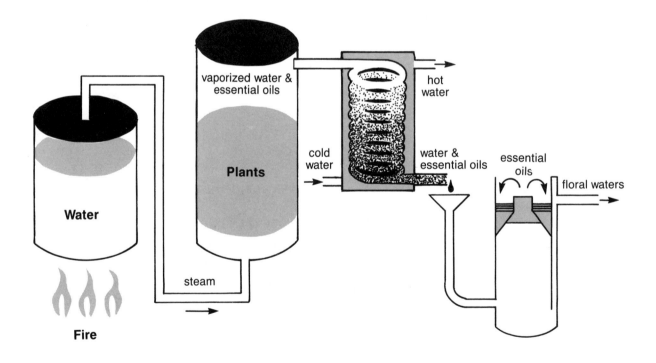

Fig. 2 The Steam Distillation Process

ies in Provence. In some areas, every village has at least one. The vats are much larger (some have up to six vats containing over 1500 gallons), and the water is now heated in a separate boiler. The people there distill mostly lavandin, a hybrid of lavender that gives a better yield of lower-quality essential oil. They also distill true lavender, hyssop, clary sage, and occasionally tarragon or cypress.

Extraction by Solvents

This relatively modern technique is used worldwide for higher yield or to obtain products that cannot be obtained by any other process. The plants are immersed in a suitable solvent (acetone or any petroleum byproduct), and the separation is performed either chemically by distillation at special temperatures that condense the oil but not the solvents. Unfortunately, such oils always contain some traces of solvent and are therefore not suitable for aromatherapy.

For the fabrication of "concretes," the material is usually soaked in hexane. The mixture is then concentrated by double distillation, and the final product has a creamy consistency due to the presence of residual solvents and waxes from the plants.

The "absolutes" are obtained from concretes by dilution in alcohol, double filtration, and double concentration, which eliminates most waxes and residual solvents.

This method is widely used for roses, neroli (orange blossoms), cassia, and tub-

eroses. It is the only way to extract the oils from jasmine, honeysuckle, carnation, and others.

Concretes and absolutes are extensively used in cosmetics and perfumery; they should not be used for aromatherapy.

Hypercritical Carbon Dioxide Extraction

Hypercritical carbon dioxide extraction is a new process that has raised great hopes among perfumers and aromatherapists. What is so hypercritical about it?

Any substance can exist in three different states: gas, liquid, and solid. Each substance may be in any of these three states depending on its temperature and pressure. In addition, certain substances can be found in the hypercritical state—that is, they are neither liquid nor gas, but rather they are both; they disperse as readily as a gas (i.e., almost instantaneously) and they have solvent properties.

At any given temperature, most substances go from gaseous at low pressure (close to vacuum for heavy substances like metal), to liquid when the pressure increases. Some substances, though, never become liquid if their temperature is maintained over their hypercritical temperature. They will instead be in the hypercritical state when pressure increases over hypercritical pressure.

Carbon dioxide (a fairly inert gas naturally occurring in the air that we breathe) has the power to become hypercritical. Even better, its hypercritical temperature is 33 °C (a little over room temperature). Hypercritical carbon dioxide then becomes an excellent solvent of fragrances and aromatic substances. The advantages are that the whole operation takes place at fairly low temperature, and therefore the fragrance is not affected by heat; the extraction is almost instantaneous (a few minutes) and is complete; and because the solvent is virtually inert, there are no chemical reactions between the solvent and the aromatic substances. In comparison, steam distillation requires 1 to 48 hours, it always leaves some residues of essential oils, and many substances are hydrolyzed or oxidized in the process.

Unlike in regular solvent extraction (concretes, absolutes, oleoresins), the solvent can be easily and totally removed, just by releasing the pressure. The whole process takes place in a closed chamber, which means that even the most volatile and most fragile fractions of the fragrance can be collected. Consequently, the end product is as close as anyone can get to the plant's aromatic substance.

Hypercritical carbon dioxide extraction then appears to be an aromatherapist's dream come true. Unfortunately, the hypercritical pressure for carbon dioxide is over 200 atmospheres (yes, 200 times the regular atmospheric pressure!), requiring very heavy and expensive stainless steel still equipment.

As far as I know, this process is still in an experimental stage. Pilot units have been built in few high-tech laboratories in France,

Germany, the United States, and Japan. (I visited the French pilot in 1987; its capacity was less than 2 gallons, whereas a regular steam still has a capacity of up to 2000 gallons.) Only small amounts of hypercritical extracts have been produced so far, but commercial production may not be too far down the line. Such products are likely to remain fairly costly for the time being.

ADULTERATIONS, PROBLEMS OF QUALITY

Most essential oils available on the market are of very poor quality for two main reasons. The first reason is that the chemical composition of the essential oils of a given plant can vary greatly, depending on the variety, the time, the soil, and the methods of cultivation and distillation. Oil of thyme, for instance, varies from 100% thymol to 90% carvacrol, with some varieties containing citral or geraniol. In addition, many of the basic components, such as linalol, cineol, borneol, citral, and nerolidol, are present in different essences. When the main components of a given essential oil are known, it is possible to reconstitute it using cheaper essential oils or their components. Rose, for instance, is often imitated with geranium, lemongrass, palmarosa, terpenic alcohol, or stearine.

The second reason is that recent advances in chemistry have flooded the market with synthetic essential oils. These synthetic reconstitutions are used mostly in the food and cosmetic industries, but also in perfumery and pharmacy. The chemicals in the oils are in perpetual interaction, and the kind of interaction depends on the way these substances are put together. The action of essential oils depends also on the processes taking place in them. Therefore, natural or synthetic reconstitutions will never replace the natural oils. For aromatherapy as well as for perfumery or cosmetics, one should only use the best quality of essential oils.

Oils extracted by cold pressure resemble most closely the products present in the plant, but only a few oils can be extracted by this method. Steam distillation yields the next best quality. I am working on a prototype of a still that incorporates recent technological advances. It will be a substantial improvement on the traditional stills and is expected to produce an even better quality of essential oils.

The oils extracted by solvents should not be used internally.

Wild plants growing in unpolluted areas or plants grown organically yield the best quality of oil. Nonorganic products are not recommended, as many synthetic pesticides are solubles in the plants' aromatic substances and may be concentrated in the oil.

FLORAL WATERS, DISTILLATES, HYDROLATES

Floral waters or hydrolates or distillates are obtained by sending steam through the plants and condensing this steam; they are often a byproduct of distillation, in which case they are recovered from the florentine vase after separation of the essential oils. The best floral waters are obtained by cohobation, a process that continuously recycles the distillate. The amount of water used for distillation is proportional to the quantity of plant; the overflow from the florentine vase is sent back into the boiler, and steam is sent through the plant material until it is saturated.

Hydrolates contain the water-soluble active principles of the plants. They retain a small amount of essential oils (about 0.2 gram/liter) that disperses in an ionized form, so that the product is less likely to cause skin irritation. They were traditionally used for skin care, for the disinfection of wounds, and for healing. Milder and easier to use than essential oils, their utility in skin care and cosmetics is considerable. Rose flower water, orange blossom water, chamomile water, and bluet water are among the most renowned.

DO IT YOURSELF

All an amateur distiller needs is a pressure cooker. Place the plants on a screen above the water. Replace the valve with a plastic hose (2 to 5 feet long), boil the water, run cold water on the hose, and collect the floral water and oils in any suitable container. You can separate the oils by decantation in glass bottles. You will not, of course, produce large amounts of oils, but their quality will be excellent and you will also obtain plenty of floral water to prepare your own cosmetics, creams, and shampoos.

I should warn you, however, that distillation is an incurable addiction. If you are genetically predisposed, you might become a distillation addict for the rest of your life!

HOW TO KEEP YOUR ESSENTIAL OILS

Essential oils are precious products that can be very expensive. (You will understand why when you start making your own.) They should be stored in tightly closed dark glass bottles to prevent their deterioration by light or by air. They should also be protected from temperature variations. Prolonged heat is not good for them.

Under normal conditions, essential oils can be considered fresh for 3 years after their extraction.

FOUR

The Chemistry of
Essential Oils

THE ATOMIC SAGA

Atoms consist of electrons, which have a negative electrical charge, orbiting around a nucleus. The nucleus contains the protons, which have a positive electrical charge, and the neutrons, with no electric charge. Each atom has the same number of electrons and protons, to bring the total electrical charge to zero. The electrons are disposed in layers around the nucleus. Each layer can hold a set maximum number of electrons. Thus, the first layer cannot contain more than two electrons, the second layer holds a maximum of eight electrons, and so on. The electrons are arranged around the nucleus so as to first fill up the innermost layers. Thus, most atoms have empty spaces in their outer layer.

Hydrogen is the most common atom in the universe and has the simplest possible structure. A single electron orbiting around one proton; it has one empty space in its single layer. Carbon, another very common atom, consists of six protons and six neutrons in the nucleus, with six orbiting electrons — two in its first layer, four in its second layer — and four empty spaces. Oxygen has eight neutrons, eight protons, and eight electrons — two in its first layer, six in its second layer — and two empty spaces.

Atoms are impelled to fill up all their electronic layers. In fact, they compusively need to fill up this outermost layer.

If they are left all alone, they usually combine with themselves. The hydrogen atoms share their electrons two by two; two oxygen atoms get together and each contribute two electrons. With carbons, things are a little bit different. Carbon atoms arrange themselves in three dimensional patterns, each carbon being attached to four other carbons and contributing one electron to each liaison. Billions of billions of carbon atoms can thus be connected in huge patterns.

But most atoms seem to prefer diversity. They combine with other atoms to form molecules in a kind of atomic mating process, called bonding. Atomic bonding consists of sharing the electrons in the outermost layer so as to fill up this layer. When two atoms share one electron in a molecular liaison, it is called a single bond. Atoms may also share two electrons in a double bond or even three electrons in a triple bond.

Hydrogen can form only a single bond; oxygen can form single bonds (as in water, where it is attached to two hydrogens) or double bonds (as in carbon dioxide, where two oxygens share two electrons each with a carbon). Carbon can also form triple bonds, usually with itself.

This is where the whole thing may turn into some kind of dreadful thriller! Quite frankly, by human standards, atomic behavior can be rather objectionable. In order to fill up their outmost layer, atoms will use any possible means. They tear molecules apart to steal other's atoms. This is called an atomic reaction. And believe me, some atomic reactions can be pretty wild. Thus, when you send, for instance, some oxygen atoms into a crowd of methane molecules (each made of four hydrogens attached to one carbon), the oxygen atoms are so anxious to combine that any spark causes an explosion. The oxygens split the methane; some oxygens get the hydrogens to create plain water, while others take care of the carbons in carbon dioxide. The whole exchange is brief but rather intense. This is

exactly what happens when a gas leak blows up a ten-story building.

When the universe was still young and reckless, the type of atomic massacre that I just described was really nothing compared to what was going on every day. As time went by, atoms settled down in more stable molecules (burned out, probably). The interchanges became more sophisticated, especially on our planet.

Molecules got bigger and bigger, until life became possible. From general warfare, atomic behavior evolved into a harmonious dance. Under the tight control of life forces, molecules go around, gently swapping atoms or atomic groups.

Carbon is the major actor in life's molecular dance. Its blatant promiscuity and its ability to link with itself allow it to generate chains of carbon atoms. In such chains, each carbon atom is linked to one (at each end of the chain) or two (inside the chain) carbon atoms. Carbons usually attach themselves to each other through a single bond. This leaves space for two or three extra bonds where hydrogen and oxygen (carbon's two major partners in life's waltz) or other radicals can be attached. Molecules as complex as DNA, life's inner memory chip, can thus be created.

The smaller molecules tend to be volatile—that is, they evaporate easily. The larger the molecule, the lower its ability to evaporate (i.e., the higher its boiling point). Essential oils are volatile; their molecules are rather small. Most of them have 10 or 15 carbon atoms (see discussion in next section of terpenoid molecules).

THE CHEMISTRY OF COMMON ESSENTIAL OILS CONSTITUENTS*

Almost all of the molecules found in essential oils are composed of carbon and hydrogen, or of carbon, hydrogen, and oxygen. The chemistry of the constituents of essential oils is determined by two factors, one artificial (the steam distillation process) and the other intrinsic to the plant (the biosynthesis of the constituent molecules).

By steam distillation, a process that is mainly physical, only volatile and water-insoluble constituents are isolated from the plant. The main types of chemical compounds isolated are terpenes and terpenoid compounds and phenylpropane-derived compounds. There are many other constituents in plants (often valuable) that do not find their way into the essential oils. Among them are all the molecules that are soluble in water, like acids or sugars, or that are too large or too high in polarity to evaporate with steam, such as tannins, flavonoids, carotenoids, and polysaccharides.

Three main categories of chemical compounds can therefore be distinguished in essential oils: (1) terpenes and terpenoid compounds; (2) sesquiterpenes and sesquiterpenoid compounds; and (3) phenylpropane derivatives. The first two share the same biosynthetic pathway.

---

* In collaboration with Kurt Schnaubelt, Ph.D.

Terpenes and Sesquiterpenes

Terpenes and sesquiterpenes are molecules made up of carbon and hydrogen (hydrocarbons). They provide the basic chemical structures through the ability of the carbon atom to form chemical bonds with other carbon atoms. Carbon atoms bonding to each other determine much of the overall shape and size of the molecule—they form the "carbon backbone" of the molecule. If the only other element present is hydrogen, the molecules are called unsubstituted and are referred to as terpenes or sesquiterpenes.

The terpenoid molecules share a common biosynthetic pathway. Their chemical structure can be looked at as if they were made up of multiples of the isoprene molecule. The isoprene structure consists of a chain of five carbon atoms. (Rationalizing the makeup of terpenoid molecules as multiples of isoprene units is a useful model, but the actual biosynthesis takes a different course.) The smallest molecules formed in this way are the monoterpenes, with 10 carbon atoms. They are the main constituents of many essential oils.

Molecules with 15 carbon atoms, sesquiterpenes, are also commonly encountered in essential oils, since they are still volatile enough to distill with steam. Molecules with 20 carbons (diterpenes) are found in essential oils to a much lesser degree. Terpenoid molecules with 30 and 40 carbon atoms also occur in plants but are not found in the essential oils. Their molecular weight is too high to allow evaporation with steam.

Important molecules of life like steroids and certain hormones are members of this last group. Monoterpenes have a 10-carbon structure, sesquiterpenes have 15 carbons, and diterpenes have 20 carbons.

Functional Groups in Essential Oils Constituents

Unsubstituted hydrocarbons can be modified by a functional group; that is, one or two hydrogen atoms are replaced by the functional group in the molecule. Within the realm of essential oils, the functional groups we have to deal with are all formed through the different ways oxygen can be attached to carbon.

Generally, molecules made up of a terpene structure and a functional group are called terpenoid (or sesquiterpenoid, from sequiterpenes). Strictly speaking, the term terpenes (or sesquiterpenes) would refer to the hydrocarbons and terpenoid to substituted terpenes. In the professional literature, the term terpene (or sesquiterpene) is often used to denote the whole group of molecules with the same basic structure, including hydrocarbons and substituted molecules.

The properties of the essential oils constituents is determined by their basic structure (mono-, sesqui-, and diterpene) and their functional group (Figure 3).

Ketones (Figure 3a)

Thujone, pulegone, pinocamphone, and carvone are important ketones. Oxygen can be attached to a carbon through a double bond. The resulting group is called a carboxyl group; if the oxygen is attached to a carbon located within a carbonic chain, the resulting molecule is called a ketone.

Monoterpenoid ketones determine the main characteristics of a fair number of essential oils, such as hyssop and sage. Other oils with a substantial ketone content are thuja and pennyroyal. The applications of these oils most relevant to aromatherapy are easing or increasing the flow of mucus and their cytophylactic effect. Both properties are utilized extensively in aromatherapy in remedies for upper respiratory complaints (mucolytic) and skin-care preparations (cytophylactic). Many ketones are neurotoxic when taken internally. Some of them can be dangerous (pulegone in pennyroyal, thujone in mugwort, *Sage officinali*, and thuja).

Aldehydes (Figure 3b)

Citral, citronellal, neral, and geranial are important aldehydes. Like ketones, aldehydes have a carboxyl group, but unlike the ketone, their oxygen is attached to a carbon that is also linked to a hydrogen, which means that they are not located within a carbonic chain.

Monoterpenoid aldehydes are the main chemical feature of the oils of melissa (*Melissa officinalis*), lemongrass, citronella, lemon verbena (*Lippia citriodora*), and *Eucalyptus* citriodora. Studies show that aldehydes found in these oils are sedative. Citral has also been found to possess strong antiseptic properties.

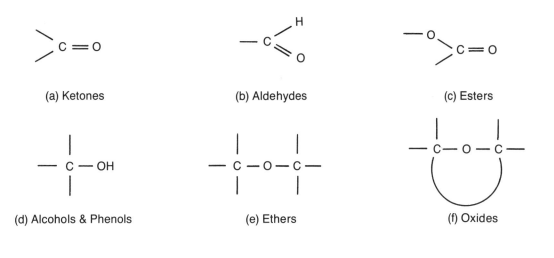

Fig. 3 Functional Groups in Essential Oil Constuents

Esters (Figure 3c)

Linalyl acetate, geranyl acetate, bornyl acetate, and methyl salicilate are important esters. Ester groups contain a double bond between carbon and oxygen (carboxyl group). A second oxygen molecule is bonded to the carboxyl group, rendering it an ester group. Esters are produced through the reaction of an alcohol and an acid. Esters are characteristically antifungal and sedative. They have a direct calming effect on the central nervous system and can be powerful spasmolytic agents.

Roman chamomile contains a number of esters that are not found commonly in other essential oils. The spasmolytic power apparently reaches a maximum in this oil.

Esters are generally fragrant and often have very fruity aromas. They are commonly used in compositions of fruit aromas and flavorings. Linalyl acetate, for instance, is found in large amounts in lavender and bergamot. It is the reaction product of linalol and acetic acid. Clary sage is another oil whose ester characteristics are obvious, especially if it is used in massage.

Esters are found in essential oils in probably larger numbers than the representatives of any of the other groups. There are not many essential oils with esters as main constituents, but often even small amounts of characteristic esters are crucial for the finer notes in the fragrance of an essential oil.

Terpene Alcohols (Figure 3d)

Linalol, borneol, citronellol, geraniol, santalol, estragol, and nerol are important alcohols. Oxygen is most often attached to a terpene molecule through a single bond in the hydroxyl group, in which a hydrogen takes up the second oxygen bond. The hydroxyl group (-O-H) consists of a water molecule (H-O-H) separated from one of its hydrogen carbons, hence its name. The hydroxyl group has very strong reactive power.

Molecules with a hydroxyl group are called alcohols. They are typically very fluid.

If an alcohol group is introduced into a terpene molecule, the resulting compound is called an alcohol or terpene alcohol. Terpene alcohols are among the most useful molecules in aromatherapy. The terpene alcohols found in common essential oils show a fair degree of diversity with respect to their properties as well as their fragrance, but also have several properties in common. Terpene alcohols are generally antiseptic, and a positive energizing effect is attributed to them. Linalol is a prominent terpene alcohol in lavender, rosewood, petitgrain, neroli, and coriander. Citronellol, which has been shown to possess antiviral qualities, is a main constituent in rose and geranium oils, and geraniol is found in palmarosa. Alpha-terpineol is characteristic in *Eucalyptus radiata* and niaouli (*Melaleuca viridiflora*). Terpineol-4 is a main constituent in tea tree and garden marjoram. Other oils also in this group are present in *Ravensare aromatica* and cajeput. All these oils have as common qualities an antiseptic nature; a pleasant, uplifting fragrance; desirable properties; and very low toxicity. The usefulness of the terpene alcohols has been pointed out again through research that suggests that those juniper oils with a high terpineol-4 content and a corresponding low content of pinenes (terpene hydrocarbons) are the safest diuretic agents among the different types of juniper oil.

Cineol (Figure 3f)

If oxygen links two carbons and at the same time is a member of a ring structure, the compound is called an oxide.

Cineol, also called eucalyptole, is almost in a class of its own. As a chemical compound it is an oxide. It imparts a strong expectorant effect to the different varieties of eucalyptus oils. It is practically ubiquitous, being a more or less desired constituent of almost every other essential oil.

Linalol oxide is an important constituent of the oil of the decumbent variety of *Hyssopus officinalis*. This oil has a low ketone content and a reduced toxicity compared with the oil of *Hyssopus officinalis*.

Phenols

Thymol, carvacrol, and eugenol are shown in Figure 4. When an alcohol hydroxyl group is attached to a benzene ring, the resulting compound is called a phenol. The phenol structure is strongly electropositive and therefore very active chemically. Phenols like thymol or carvacrol are the strongest antibacterial agents among the mono-

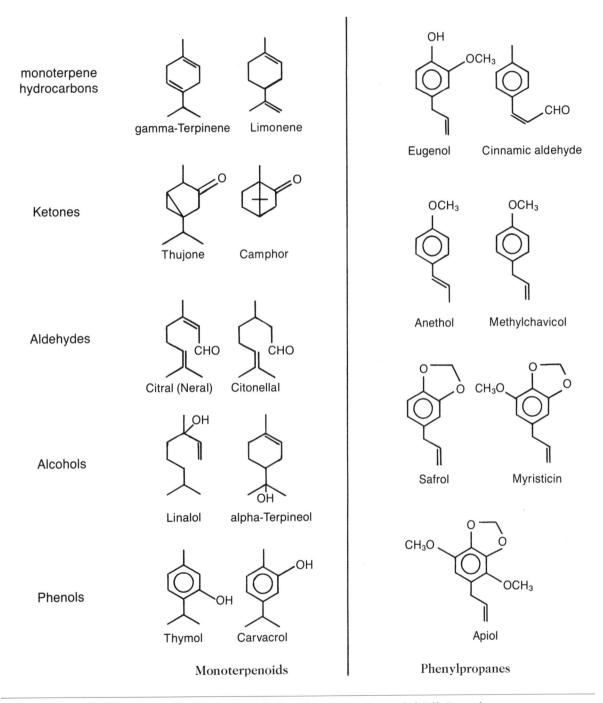

monoterpene
hydrocarbons

gamma-Terpinene   Limonene

Ketones

Thujone   Camphor

Aldehydes

Citral (Neral)   Citonellal

Alcohols

Linalol   alpha-Terpineol

Phenols

Thymol   Carvacrol

Monoterpenoids

Eugenol   Cinnamic aldehyde

Anethol   Methylchavicol

Safrol   Myristicin

Apiol

Phenylpropanes

Fig. 4 Examples of Terpene and Phenylpropane Essential Oil Constituents

terpenoid compounds of aromatherapy.

Their strongly stimulant character is widely utilized in aromatherapy; however, these oils can be very irritating and they should be used only in appropriately low concentrations.

Phenylpropane Derivatives

Eugenol, cinnamic aldehyde, anethol, methylchavicol, safrol, myristicin, and apiol are shown in Figure 4 (also see Table 1). The common characteristic of this class of essential oil constituents is that they are all derived from the phenylpropane structure. The elements that make up this structure are an "aromatic" phenyl ring system with a propane (three-carbon) side chain. This basic structure of nine carbon atoms is then modified by various groups attached to it. A double bond in the side chain often allows the attached groups to interact with the pi-electron system of the aromatic ring, rendering some molecules in this group pharmacologically highly active. Their biosynthetic pathway, originating through shikimic acid, is different from those of the terpenoids.

Cinnamon and clove, like the phenolic essences, are strong antiseptic agents. They can cause severe skin reactions and must be used with caution. Eugenol, the main constituent of clove oil, besides being antiseptic and fungicidal, shows local anesthetic properties. It has also been reported to inhibit certain carcinogenic processes. The same effect was found for caryophyllen, another constituent of clove oil (see sesquiterpenes). Aniseed, basil, and tarragon are not as aggressive as cinnamon or clove can be; yet they all share a distinctly sweet

Table 1. Properties of Phenylpropane-Derived Essential Oil Constituents

Phenylpropane derivative	Property	Source
Eugenol Cinnamic aldehyde	Antiseptic Stimulant Skin irritants	Clove Cinnamon
Anethol Methylchavicol	Increase secretion Expectorant Spasmolytic	Aniseed Basil, tarragon Parsley, nutmeg, sassafras
Safrol, myristicin, apiol	Diuretic Spasmolytic Abortive (apiol) Central nervous system stimulant Hallucinogenic (myristicin)	

Table 2. Properties of Terpenoid Essential Oil Constituents

Terpenoid	Property	Source
Ketones	Promote tissue formation Mucolytic Potentially neurotoxic	Sage, thuja, wormwood (thujone), hyssop (pinocamphone)
Aldehydes	Antiinflammative Sedative Antiviral	Melissa, lemongrass (citrals), citronella, *Eucalyptus citriodora* (citronellal)

Terpene alcohols	Bactericidal
	Toning
	Diuretic
	Antiviral
		Lavender, coriander, petitgrain,
		    rosewood (linalol),
		    Eucalyptus radiata, niaouli (alpha[terpineol),
		    tea tree, marjoram, juniper (terpineol-4)

Esters	Spasmolytic
	Sedative
	Can be antifungal
		Roman chamomile (angelica acid esters)
		    lavender, clary sage, bergamot (linalyl
		    acetate)

Cineol	Expectorant	Eucalyptus and many other oils
Phenols	Bactericidal Immunostimulant Stimulant Skin irritant Potentially toxic to liver	Thyme (thymol), oregano, savory (carvacrol)

character in their fragrance. The main constituents of basil and anise seed oils, methylchavicol and anethol, can cause negative effects if used in unreasonably high concentrations. Others in this group include safrol (sassafras, camphor), myristicin (nutmeg), and apiol (parsley). While most of these oils can be beneficially used in aromatherapy, they share a potential for toxicity in high concentrations or with prolonged use. The potential of nutmeg to act as a hallucinogen (dosages required to induce these effects are unsafe and can cause lasting damage or death), and the effects of anethol, well known through its abuses in anise liqueurs, demonstrate the ability of phenylpropane constituents to interact with the central nervous system in a way that depends strongly on dosage and/or concentration.

Many of the properties of terpenoid essential oil constituents (ketones, aldehydes, terpene alcohols, esters, cineol, and phenols) are listed in Table 2.

Table 3. General Effects of Terpenoid Compounds*

Activity	Monoterpenes	Sesquiterpenes	Diterpenes
Anesthetic	+		
Analeptic	+	+	
Analgestic		+	
Anthelmintic	+	+	
Antiarrythmic		+	
Antibiotic (antibacterial, antifungal, antiseptic, antiviral)	+	+	+
Antiepileptic		+	
Antihistaminic	+		
Antiinflammatory, antiphlogistic	+	+	
Antirheumatic	+		
Antitumor (antiblastic, anticarcinogenic, cytotoxic)	+	+	+
Choleretic, cholagogue		+	
Diuretic	+		
Expectorant	+		+
Hypotensive	+	+	+
Insecticidal	+		+
Irritant	+	+	
Juvenile hormone		+	
Pheromone	+	+	
Phytohormone (growth regulating)		+	+
Purgative	+		+
Sedative	+	+	
Spasmolytic	+	+	
Toxic		+	+
Vitamin			+

*The biological, pharmacological, and therapeutical activity of normal monoterpenes (and also of many sesquiterpenes) is closely connected to that of the essential oils. An overview of the most important biological properties of mono-, sesqui- and diterpenes is given here.

Terpene Hydrocarbons

Limonene (present at 90% or more in most citrus oils), pinene, camphene, and myrcene are shown in Figure 4. With regard to their properties, terpene hydrocarbons are often thought to be rather insignificant constituents of essential oils. There has been discussion of whether terpenes are skin or mucous membrane irritants. Studies of various pine oils show that antiseptic principles are formed when these oils are subjected to natural or induced aging or oxidation. A study of the effects of terpenes against Herpes simplex and other viruses should renew the respect for terpenes in aromatherapy.

Limonene, the main constituent of many citrus oils; alpha-sabinene; and gamma-terpinene have all been found to possess antiviral properties. Essential oils with high proportions of monoterpene hydrocarbons include:

> Lemon, orange, bergamot (limonene)
> Black pepper (pinenes, camphenes, etc.)
> Pine oils (pinenes)
> Turpentine (pinenes, limonene)
> Nutmeg (pinenes)
> Mastick (pinenes)
> Angelica (pinenes)

Table 3 illustrates the activities of monoterpenes, as well as sesquiterpenes and diterpenes.

Sesquiterpenes

Chamazulen, bisabolol, santalol, zingiberol, carotol, caryophyllen, and farnesol are among the important sesquiterpenes. Table 4 lists some sources of sesquiterpenes.

As we look at sesquiterpene constituents of essential oils, the influence of a functional group becomes less dominating. The increased size of the overall structure brings about increased complexity. The interaction between carbon backbone and functional group becomes more subtle and intricate. The individuality of the molecule becomes a greater factor in the makeup of the pharmacological effect of the molecule.

More than 2000 sesquiterpenes have been isolated from plants to date, and their

Table 4. Sources of Sesquiterpenes in Essential Oils

Sesquiterpene	Property	Source
		From roots
Zingiberol		Ginger
Vetiveron, vetiverol	Stomachic, carminative	Vetiver
Complex composition (almost 100% sesquiterpenes)		Spikenard
Valeranon (valepotriates C 101)	Sedative, spasmolytic	Valerian
		From wood, seeds, or leaves
Alpha-santalol		Sandalwood
Patchouli alcohol		Patchouli
Carotol		Carrot seed
Nerolidol (dependent on type)	Disinfectant Antiseptic	Niaouli
		From the plant family asteraceae
Chamazulene, bisabolol	Antiphlogistic	German chamomile
Chamazulene (dependent on chemotype)		Yarrow
Chamazulene (dependent on chemotype)		Tansy

structures vary widely. Most of these sesquiterpenes can be attributed to 30 main structural types. A summary of their biological activity is shown in Table 5.

Essential oils with a high proportion of sesquiterpene constituents are mostly distilled from roots and woods or from plants of the Asteraceae family.

Sesquiterpenes have been the object of much interest and research into their properties. The bulk of that research has been performed on sesquiterpenes isolated from plants of the Asteraceae family that are not common essential oil plants. The situation for the aromatherapist is somewhat unsatisfactory, since there are good reasons to speculate on the potential properties of sesquiterpenes in essential oils, but only limited availability of substantiating research data. There are some notable exceptions. In the effort to provide a scientific basis for the many uses of German chamomile (*Chamomilla matricaria*), the antiphlogistic properties of chamazulene and alpha-bisabolol were firmly established.

Farnesol is a sesquiterpene whose superior properties as a bacteriostatic and dermatophilic agent are well documented. Because of its ability to inhibit the growth of bacteria rather than killing them, it is an ideal deodorizing agent, since it inhibits the development of odor-causing microorganisms without eliminating the bacteria that are present on healthy skin.

Finally, caryophyllen, which is found in many essential oils, most notably in clove oil, has received renewed attention. It combines sedative and antiviral effects with an ability to inhibit some carcinogenic processes.

Sandalwood illustrates the lack of solid research data on sesquiterpenes that are found in essential oils. On one hand there is ample anecdotal evidence for its usefulness in urinary tract infections, and even pharmacological textbooks list it as a poten-

Table 5. Sesquiterpenes from Essential Oils with Known Pharmacological Properties

Sesquiterpene	Property	Source
Chamazulene	Antiphlogistic Antiinflammatory	German chamomile, yarrow, tansy
Caryophyllen	Sedative Antiviral Potentially anticarcinogenic	Clove (10%); occurs in many essential oils in low concentrations
Farnesol	Bacteriostatic	Rose, chamomile, and many other flower oils

tial urine disinfectant. On the other hand, an antibacterial effect of the sandalwood oil constituents has not been confirmed. It is of course tempting to speculate that searching for an outright bactericidal effect of santalol may be the wrong experiment in light of the fact that sesquiterpenes can be effective immune stimulants. The effect of the oil could be caused not through direct bactericidal action but rather through stimulation of the body's defense mechanisms.

A summary of essential oils and their major chemical components is given in Table 6.

Table 6. Essential Oils and Their Major Chemical Components

Plant	Number of carbons	Components
Angelica	10	Musk ketone
Aniseed	9	Phenylpropane: *trans*-anethole
Basil	9	Phenylpropane: methylchavicol
Bay		Phenylpropanes: myrcene, eugenol, charvicol
Bergamot	10	Terpenes and esters: limonene, linalyl acetate
Birch		Esters: methyl salicilate
Cajeput	10	Terpene alcohols: alpha-Terpineol
Caraway	10	Ketones: limonene, carvone
Cardamom	10	Terpenes: cineole
Carrot seed	15	Sesquiterpene alcohol: carotol
Cedarwood		Ketone: atlantone-7
Chamomile, blue		Sesquiterpinoids: chamazulene
Chamomile, German	15	Sesquiterpinoids: bisabolol, chamazulene
Chamomile, mixta		Alcohol: ormenol
Chamomile, Roman		Esters
Cinnamon bark	9	Phenylpropane: cinnamic aldehyde
Cinnamon leaf	9	Phenylpropane: eugenol
Cistus		Terpenes
Citronella	10	Aldehydes: citronellal
Clary sage		Esters: linalyl acetate
Clove buds	9	Phenylpropane: eugenol
Coriander seeds		Terpene alcohols: linalool
Cumin seeds		Aldehyde: cuminaldehyde
Cypress	10	Terpenes: terpenyl acetate
Elemi	10	Terpenes: limonene, elemol
Eucalyptus australiana		Cineole
Eucalyptus citriodora		Aldehydes: citronellal
Eucalyptus globulus	10	Cineole, *t*-alcohol

Table 6. (continued)

Plant	Number of carbons	Components
Everlasting		Esters: neryl esters
Fennel		Phenylpropane: *trans*-anethole
Fir	10	Terpenes
Frankincense	10	Terpenes: phellandrene, camphene, olibanol
Geranium	10	Alcohols: citronellol, geraniol
Ginger root	15	Sesquiterpenoids: zingiberone
Grapefruit	10	Terpenes: limonene
Hyssop	10	Ketone: pinocarvone
Jasmine		Benzyl acetate, jasmone
Juniper	10	Terpenes, terpene alcohol
Laurel	10	Cineole
Lavender	10	Esters, terpene alcohols: linalyl acetate
Lavandin	10	Esters, terpene alchols: linalol, camphor, linalyl acetate
Lemon	10	Terpenes, aldehyde: limonene, citral
Lemongrass	10	Aldehydes: citral
Lime	10	Terpenes, aldehyde: limonene, citral
Litsea cubeba	10	Aldehyde: citrals
Lovage root		Lactones
Marjoram	10	Terpene alcohols: terpine-4-ol
Marjoram, wild Spanish	10	Phenol
Melissa	10	Aldehyde: citrals
Mugwort	10	Ketone: thujone
Myrrh	10	Terpenes
Myrtle	10	Terpenes, terpene alcohols
Neroli	10	Terpene alcohols, esters: linalool, geraniol, nerol
Niaouli	10	Terpenes, terpene alcohols
Nutmeg	9	Terpenes, alcohols: linalol, borneol, myristicine
Orange	10	Terpenes
Oregano	10	Phenol: carvacrol
Palmarosa	10	Terpene alcohols: geraniol
Patchouli	15	Sesquiterpenoids: patchoulol
Pennyroyal	10	Ketone: pulegone, menthone
Pepper	10	Terpenes: piperine
Peppermint	10	Terpene alcohols: menthol, carvone, linalool
Petitgrain biguarade	10	Terpenes, esters: linalyl acetate
Pine	10	Terpenes
Rose	10	Alcohols: citronellol, geraniol, nerol
Rosemary	10	Terpenes, terpene alcohols: cineole
Rosewood	10	Terpene alcohols: linalool
Sage lavandulifolia	10	Cineole, camphor, esters

Table 6. (continued)

Plant	Number of carbons	Components
Sandalwood, Mysore	15	Sesquiterpenoids: santalol
Savory	10	Phenol: carvacrol
Spearmint	10	Terpene alcohols: carvone
Spike	10	Terpene alcohols: linalool, camphor
Spruce	10	Terpenes
Tangerine	10	Terpenes
Tarragon	9	Phenylpropane: methylchavicol
Tea tree	10	Terpenes, terpene alcohols: terpinen-4-ol
Therebentine	10	Terpenes: p-menthadienes
Thyme, citriodora		Aldehyde: citral
Thyme, lemon		Alcohol: linalool
Thyme, red		Phenol: thymol
Verbena, lemon	10	Aldehyde: citrals
Vetiver	15	Sesquiterpenoids: vetiveron, vetiverol
Ylang ylang		Alcohols: geraniol, linalol, ylangol

FIVE

How to Use Essential Oils

Essential oils are highly concentrated plant extracts and very potent medicines that should not be abused. Each drop is equivalent to at least 1 ounce of plant material. Therefore, it is always important to use exact doses and to recall that in most cases, essential oils are more potent at infinitesimal doses.

Essential oils can be used (a) internally (by ingestion), (b) externally through the skin (massage, bath, friction, application), (c) for skin care and cosmetic use (facials, compresses, masks, lotions, creams), (d) for hair care, and (e) through the respiratory system (inhalation, nebulization). They can also be injected, but this must be strictly confined to medical practice.

Whether taken internally or externally, essential oils diffuse through the skin and membranes and penetrate deeply into the tissues and the circulatory system. Therefore, external application is a very efficient way to treat specific organs. As a rule, ingestion is recommended for infectious diseases and for action on the digestive system (throat, stomach, liver, etc.), although a massage of the corresponding zone is very helpful in such cases.

The nebulizer probably provides the most convenient way to take essential oils. It is recommended for all diseases related to the lungs, the heart, the brain, and the blood.

INTERNAL USE

Essential oils can be taken undiluted on a small piece of sugar or mixed with honey. In this case, it is very important to carefully use exact doses. Any oil can be dangerous at high doses; the most toxic are, in decreasing order, rue, thuja, mugwort, *Sage officinalis*, hyssop, anise, and fennel.

As a rule, whenever essential oils are taken internally, the maximum dose should be 5 drops three times a day.

For a more flexible and convenient internal use, essential oils can be diluted in ethyl alcohol (or sweet almond oil for children and people intolerant to alcohol). Mix 1/4 oz. essential oils (either a single oil or a blend) in 4 oz. of 90% ethyl alcohol (do not use rubbing alcohol). The average dose is 25 drops, three times a day in a glass of warm water or herb tea, between meals. Maximum dose: 150 drops a day.

Aromatic honey:

1/4 oz. of your blend of essential oils in 16 oz honey.
Stir thoroughly.
Dose: 1/2 teaspoon three times a day.
A more concentrated preparation can be made for use in capsules.

<u>**Contraindications:**</u> Heartburn, ulcers.

EXTERNAL USE

While essential oils are only taken internally for therapeutic purposes, they can be used externally for their pleasurable aspects and for well-being. Like spices in food, they add a touch of taste, genuineness, and elegance to existence. In acute conditions, the pleasure that they provide is at least as important as their strictly therapeutic effects.

Massage

Essential oils are particularly beneficial in massage—a slow, diffuse, gentle, and pleasant way to take them. They are completely absorbed by the skin in 60 to 120 minutes and penetrate deeply into the tissues. In a way they act like natural implants. By their prolonged action, they amplify the effects of the massage itself. Hand healing and massage are probably the most ancient healing arts. The ancients used oils for massage, usually scented oils.

Massage goes much further than a mere tissue manipulation. It is a direct and simple form of communication between the masseur or masseuse and the patient in which the hands are extremely sensitive receptors. During the course of the massage, the hands discover the internal geography of the body, unraveling tensions, sores, hidden pains, sensitive points, congested areas, and swollen parts, and they tell a lot about the patient. This is why, in order to give the full benefit of a massage, the masseur or masseuse must be in an open, understanding, and compassionate state of mind.

In massage, the hands are channels of healing energy; they heal at the physical, emotional, and psychic levels. Therefore, aromatherapy massage is an excellent therapeutic combination, as essential oils and massage have mutually enhancing effects. The massage itself helps the penetration of the oils into the tissues and directs them where they are the most needed. They act locally or via the energy channels (nerves, meridians).

How to Prepare a Massage Oil

Always use cold-pressed oils as the base of your massage oil. Sweet almond oil is the most commonly used. Although they are rather new on the American market, grapeseed and canola oils are increasingly popular among massage therapists and beauticians.

For dry skin, use almond, castor, cocoa butter, olive, palm, or peanut oils.

For normal skin, use corn, cottonseed, sesame, sunflower, grapeseed, or canola oils.

For oily skin, use linseed, soybean, or most nut oils.

A small amount of wheat germ oil will bring some vitamins to the skin and will act as a natural antioxidant.

Mix 1/4 oz. of a blend of essential oil in 12-14 oz. of vegetable oil (for instance, 4 oz. sweet almond, 4 oz. safflower, 4 oz. avocado, 2 oz. wheat germ, 2 oz. sesame).

Calming massage oil:
Marjoram, orange, lavender, fir, chamomile, vegetable oil.
Neroli or ylang ylang may also be added.
Will induce a deep relaxation of the tissues, muscles and joints and reestablish a good balance of energy.

Aphrodisiac massage oil:
Cedarwood, geranium, ylang ylang, vetiver, clary sage, pepper, cistus, sandalwood, vegetable oil. A delightful prelude or interlude.

Pain reliever:
Birch, rosemary, lavender, thyme, pine, camomile, vegetable oil.

Also: peppermint, camphor, juniper, ginger, nutmeg.
Rheumatic crisis neuralgia, sores, and muscular aches.

Tonic massage oil:
Lemon, peppermint, pennyroyal, sage, thyme, oregano, vegetable oil.
Ginger, nutmeg, pepper, ylang ylang may also be used.
General tonic of the endocrine glands and nervous system. To tone the tissue (energetic massage).

Circulation:
Cypress, geranium, lemon, thyme, vegetable oil.
Strengthen the circulatory system (lymphatic system, capillaries and veins) and liquify the blood. For varicosis, hemorrhoids, obesity.
In case of herpes crisis, massage the inflamed area.

These oils (especially the circulation oil) can be used after the bath to moisturize and soften the skin. Different oils can be used for different parts of the body, espcially for a desired action on other organs. Refer to the therapeutic guide for more specific preparations.

Aromatic Baths

From Egypt to India, the ancients had elaborate ritual ablutions that were combinations of hot and cold baths, ointments, and aromatic massages. Essential oils and baths have synergistic effects. They enhance the pleasure of the bath and, to quote Robert Tisserand, "If they please the nose, they also please the spirit. Then there is the physiological action of the essences on the nervous system and the rest of the body." You can use the oils pure, diluted in liquid soap or alcohol, or mixed with vegetable oil (recommended for dry skin: use sweet almond, wheat germ, or avocado).

Pour the oils in your bath just before getting in to avoid an early evaporation of the oils, using 5 to 15 drops of essences in a normal bath. I strongly recommend using a dispersant for your bath preparations to avoid possible skin irritations. Aroma Vera Inc. (see resource guide) offers a line of carriers (vegetable oils and foaming bath gel base) for this purpose.

A thin film of oil will envelop your body delightfully when you slip into your bath, and will penetrate your skin and diffuse into the tissues. Relax, enjoy.

Calming bath (evening): Lavender, marjoram, chamomile

Stimulant (morning): Sage, rosemary, pine.

Aphrodisiac: Ylang ylang, sandalwood, ginger, peppermint, pepper, savory.

Lungs: Eucalyptus, lavender, pine, cajuput, copaiba, hyssop.

Rheumatic pains and muscular aches: Birch, juniper, rosemary, thyme, vetiver, sassafras.

Nervousness: Mugwort, petitgrain, marjoram, neroli.

See the therapeutic guide for more specific indications.

SKIN CARE, COSMETIC USES

Applied to the skin, essential oils regulate the activity of the capillaries and restore vitality to the tissues. According to Marguerite Maury (*The Secret of Life and Youth*), they are natural rejuvenating agents. They facilitate the elimination of waste matter and dead cells and promote the regeneration of new, healthy cells (cytophylactic power). The most pleasant scents (especially flower oils) are the most useful for skin care. They can be used in facial steam baths, compresses, masks, and body wraps. They can be added to any kind of lotion, skin cream, gel, toilet water, or perfume.

Start your skin care session with a massage of the face and the neck to activate the capillary circulation and open the pores.

Then clean the skin with a cleansing lotion, facial steam bath, compress, or mask. (People with acne rosacea or a blotchy complexion should not use steam baths or masks, as this increases the circulation and may cause more broken capillaries.)

Finally, close the pores (using compresses with cypress, juniper, or bergamot) and protect your skin with a moisturizing cream or oil (aloe vera gel with a few drops of essential oils, for instance).

As a rule, never apply essential oils undiluted on the skin.

Essential Oils for Skin Care

General skin care: Chamomile, carrot, geranium, lavender, lemon, ylang ylang.

Normal skin: Clary sage, geranium, lavender, ylang ylang.

Dry skin: Peppermint, clary sage, rosemary, sandalwood, rose, palmarosa, carrot.

Oily skin: Lavender, lemon, geranium, basil, camphor, frankincense, cedarwood, ylang ylang.

Watery skin (skin with a tendency to retain water): Lavender, rosemary, juniper, lemon.

Inflamed skin: Chamomile, clary sage, geranium, lavender, lemon, myrrh, patchouli, carrot, floral waters.

Sensitive skin: Chamomile, neroli, floral water.

Acne: Cajuput, bergamot, eucalyptus, juniper, lavender, palmarosa, niaouli.

Eczema: Cedarwood, chamomile, lavender, sage, patchouli, rose.

Rejuvenation: Chamomile, benzoin, frankincense, cedarwood, geranium, lavender, myrrh, rosemary, carrot.

Seborrhea: Bergamot, lavender, cypress, patchouli.

Wrinkles: Fennel, lemon, palmarosa, myrrh frankincense, patchouli, clary sage, carrot.

Sun photosynthesis (increases suntan): Bergamot.

Note: Floral waters are particularly suited to skin care. Milder and easier to use than essential oils, they are recommended for sensitive and inflamed skins.

Essential oils and floral water have more or less the same indications. Plain floral water can be used for compresses and should be used instead of water in any skin care preparation.

Finally, floral water in a spray bottle (rose, sage, rosemary, lavender, cypress, etc.) provides an excellent refreshing facial tonic and astringent.

Facial Steam Bath

Use 5 to 15 drops of oil in a bowl of hot water; cover your head with a large towel and let the steam unclog your pores. Add a few drops every 5 minutes (10-15 minutes all together.)

Facial Compresses

Use 5 drops of the appropriate blend of oils in a bowl of warm water. Soak cotton or cloth, apply to your face for 5 minutes, resoak, and reapply up to three times.

Masks

Facial masks are cleansing, nourishing, and revitalizing; they promote the elimination of waste material and stimulate local blood circulation. They can also be soothing and moisturizing, depending on the ingredients.

Basic ingredients are clay, oatmeal, fruits or vegetables, vegetable oil, floral water, and essential oils. Put a few spoonfuls of clay and soaked oatmeal in a bowl; add the fruit (or vegetable) pulp and juice, and slowly add a teaspoon of vegetable oil (wheat germ, for instance) and 5 drops of essential oils. Stir and add floral water, herb tea, or plain water until the mixture has the right consistency.

Apply on your face with the fingertips and let dry for up to 15 minutes, then gently take it off with a wet sponge. Apply floral water to close the pores. Normal skin needs a mask every 1 to 2 weeks.

Besides oatmeal, clay, essential oils, and floral water, you can use, for special conditions:

Acne: cabbage, grape, yeast

Oily skin: cabbage, cucumber, lemon, grape, pear, strawberry

Dry skin: melon, carrot, avocado, wheat germ oil

Sensitive skin: honey, apple, grape, melon

Mature skin: apple, avocado, wheat germ oil

Normal skin: avocado, lemon, peach, wheat germ oil

Aromatic Body Wrap

Place a blanket on a comfortable horizontal surface (bed, carpet, or massage table.) Cover the blanket with plastic and place a large towel on top.

Mix 10 to 15 drops of the appropriate blend of essential oils with 8 to 12 oz. of hot water in a spray bottle. Some aromatherapy suppliers, such as Aroma Vera Inc, offer a line of "aromasols" (blends of essential oils in an emulsifier), which allow an easier and faster dispersion of the oils in the water. Shake well. Spray the mixture on the towel, shaking the bottle constantly. Lie on the towel and wrap it around your whole body; then wrap the plastic and the blanket around your body.

Breathe, relax, enjoy. . . even better in a

quiet room with dim light and nice, peaceful music.

Lotions, Potions, Body Oils, Bath Oils, Ointments: From Cleopatra to Mary Magdalene

Numerous stories, from the remotest antiquity to the Renaissance, from the Holy Bible to the most lascivious oriental tales, seem to exude the intriguing fragrances of scented ointments or potions. Mary Magdalene gave a foot rub to Christ with precious ointments. According to venomous tongues, Cleopatra owed her seductive power to her secret potions rather than to her beauty. And so the stories continue.

Lotions, potions, creams, and ointments have the following basic ingredients:

A solidifier (lanolin or beeswax)
An oil (sweet, almond, avocado, olive, cocoa... check under "massage oil" to determine which vegetable oil to use for your type of skin)
Distillates or flower water (or distilled water)
A blend of essential oils (see under skin care)

The product that results will depend on the proportion of the ingredients (for a cream: 1 oz. beeswax, 4 oz. vegetable oil, 2 oz. water 1/4 oz. essential oils).

Melt the solidifier in a double saucepan, then slowly add the oil and water, stirring continuously. Let the mixture cool a bit until it starts to thicken, then add the essential oils and stir thoroughly. Store in tightly closed opaque jars.

HAIR CARE

Mix 1/4 oz. of essential oil in 16 oz. of a good shampoo or hair conditioner.

Scalp rub: Flower waters or:
1/4 oz. essential oils in 4 oz. grain alcohol or sweet almond oil.

Dry hair: Cade, cedarwood.

Hair loss: Cedarwood, juniper, lavender, rosemary, sage.

Normal hair: Chamomile, lavender, ylang ylang.

Oily hair: Lemongrass, rosemary

Scalp diseases: Cedarwood, rosemary, sage, cade.

Dandruff: Rosemary, cedarwood, cade.

AROMATIC DIFFUSION, INHALATION

The use of aromatic fumigations is probably as old as humanity. Priests, sorcerers, and healers of all traditions have used them extensively in their ceremonies and various rituals. Ancient Egyptians burned perfumes in the streets and inside the temples. More than 2000 years ago, Hippocrates, the father of Western medicine, successfully struggled against the epidemic of plague in Athens, using aromatic fumigations throughout the city. In the Middle Ages, people burned pine or other fragrant woods in the streets in time of epidemic to cast out devils. Perfumers were known to be resistant to diseases.

Nowadays, technology has developed a new process that does not have the inconvenience of smoke. Coming from Europe, where it is quite popular in the natural therapy movement, the aromatic diffuser disperses essential oils in the air without altering or heating them. It projects drops of essential oils in a Pyrex nebulizer, using air as a propellant. The nebulizer acts as an expansion chamber where the drops of oil are broken into a very thin mist. Since air is the gas propellant, there is no chemical pollution, no alteration of the oils, and no decomposition by heat. The ionized microparticles, which stay suspended for several hours, revitalize the air by their antiseptic and deodorant action. The oxidation of the essential oils provokes the formation of low doses of natural ozone, which decomposes in ionic nascent oxygen. This process, occurring naturally in forests, has an invigorating and purifying effect.

Clinical research on the use of this apparatus over the last 10 years shown that a thinner diffusion gives better results. Besides the antiseptic action, already widely documented, there is a very strong action on the lungs and the respiratory system in general, providing relief for asthma, bronchitis, cold, sinusitis, sore throats, etc. The action on the circulatory system, the heart, and the nervous system is also very pronounced.

In fact, the aromatic diffuser can be used for almost all the prescriptions of aromatherapy. It is the subtlest, easiest, and most pleasant way to take essential oils.

Many naturopathic and yoga centers use this apparatus in France. It can be installed in any public or private place where air treatment is needed: saunas, hot tubs, hospitals, consulting rooms, waiting rooms, gymnastic centers, schools, and of course at home—in the living room, bedroom, kitchen, or bath.

There is an obvious connection between the psychic centers and the lungs. Most spiritual practices emphasize the importance of breathing. The aromatic diffuser is then the best way to experience the subtle effects of essential oils and their effects on the spirit and the soul. By contributing to a cheerful atmosphere, it enhances the quality of life, giving it a taste of natural elegance. It is thus a precious tool for the holistic practitioner.

Some Oils to Use in the Diffuser

The sense of smell is very subjective. We particularly like some fragrances and dislike others, depending on so many factors that it is impossible to tell which ones will be our favorites. Besides, our appreciation depends on our mood, the time of the day, the season, and so on. I will give a general description of the uses of fragrance for individual oils.

Calming (evening): Lavender, marjoram, chamomile.

Stimulant (morning): Sage, rosemary, pine, mints.

Aphrodisiac: Ylang ylang, sandalwood, ginger, peppermint, pepper, savory.

Lungs: Eucalyptus, lavender, pine, cajuput, copaiba, hyssop.

Nervousness: Mugwort, petitgrain, marjoram, neroli.

Hypertension: Ylang ylang, lavender, lemon, marjoram.

Hypotension: Hyssop, sage, thyme, rosemary.

Antidepressants: Frankincense, myrrh, cedarwood.

Purifier: Lavandin, lemongrass, lemon, pine, chamomile, geranium, oregano.

Revivifier: Pine, fir, black spruce.

To strengthen the brain and fortify memory: Basil, juniper, rosemary.

Insomnia: Neroli, marjoram, chamomile.

See the therapeutic guide for more indications.

CONCLUSION

When you first step into the world of essences, you may be a little surprised or even slightly turned off. Your olfactory system will have to be reeducated, or rather detoxified. After years of neglect and abuse with inferior perfumes, your nose may not be able to fully appreciate the richness of natural fragrances. Likewise, when you change your eating habits from junk food to a more healthy diet, you cannot really appreciate the full flavor of a lettuce leaf, a plain radish, or a bowl of brown rice. But when you start to detoxify, your taste improves and becomes refined, and soon you do not want to return to junk food again.

Then fragrances reveal their power to you every day; you play with them, dance with them, create with them. They connect you to the quintessence of the realm of plants and will "make thee glad, merry, gracious and well-beloved of all men."

SIX

The Essential Oils

Plants are classified in botanical families according to the structure of their flowers. This classification goes beyond the flower itself, and each plant of the same family appears like a variation of the basic model of the type: same leaf and seed structure, similar rhythm (in space and time), similar chemical composition.

With Goethe, the anthroposophists believe in an archetypal plant that exhibits the structural potentialities of the vegetable kingdom and manifests itself through different degrees of differentiation in families, species, and chemotypes. In this system, each type expressed by the botanical families represents a certain degree of evolution of the archetypal model—a certain level of actualization of its potentialities, from the primitive equisetaceae (horsetail) to the most evolved rosaceae (rose, apple, etc.). Differentiation of the type generates the species (or genus), which is then further

differentiated in subspecies and chemotypes.

In the anthroposophic vision, inspired by the works of Paracelsus and the study of homeopathy, the physical aspect of the plants and the nature of their interactions with the environment are correlated with their medicinal properties. A type of therapeutic activity is attributed to each botanical family, variations being related to each plant of the family. This approach is quite rich and accurate. It is fairly consistent with the more classical systems of herbal therapy and aromatherapy: there are some obvious similarities between the recommended uses of plants in the same family.

While a wildcrafter in southern France, I experienced the accuracy of such a vision. In some powerful experiences of intimate communication with plants, I felt that the plants introduced themselves to me and I could tell the medicinal properties or even the names of plants that I had never seen before. More generally, I found that careful observation of the plant and its environment told me much about its activity.

At any rate, classification of essential oils by botanical families tells more about their therapeutic activity than a mere alphabetical classification, and that will be my approach in this chapter. I hope that this will give my readers a better understanding of aromatherapy.

SYNTHETICS VERSUS NATURAL: DOES IT MAKE SCENTS?

Many people think that molecules produced through the processes of life are more active in a living context (such as medicine) than their synthetic counterparts are, although they cannot really be chemically differentiated from their natural cousins. There is even growing evidence that this belief is well founded. Along the same line of thought, a natural extract is often found to be more efficient than its main active ingredient.

Could it be that molecules have some kind of memory? That they store the information pertaining to their history? That life shares a common pool of memories? That natural molecules are more accurate in dealing with living organisms because they have stored living memory?

If this is true, a natural molecule could "know" how to deal with other living molecules. Each molecule belonging to a given

extract would have a memory of its companions and could predictably be more efficient when not separated from these companions.

The Concept of Morphogenetic Field

When bicycles were first invented, it took people months to learn how to ride them. How long did it take your kids to learn how to ride their bikes? A few hours? Two days?

When the first cars were invented, most people were too scared to even think about driving them. Now the average teenager learns how to drive in almost no time.

When Einstein introduced the theory of relativity, years passed before a handful of people could figure it out. Nowadays, relativity is taught in college.

How long did it take you to learn how to use a computer? How long did it take your kids?

When you look at up-to-date college textbooks, how often do you feel that you haven't any clue to what they are all about?

According to Rupert Sheldrake, all these phenomena can be accounted for by the concept of morphogenetic fields.

To put it simply, a morphogenetic field can be viewed as a landscape, with mountains, valleys, plains, riverbeds, and so on. Each valley, each riverbed corresponds to flows of information, all interconnected. A totally new input of information can be viewed as a small furrow being traced somewhere in the landscape. The more this information is used, the deeper its furrow becomes, and the more likely it will be to attract new information, until it resembles a valley, or a main stream. Learning a new technique, for instance, deepens the corresponding furrow. The more people learn this technique, the deeper the furrow, and the easier it becomes for other people to learn the technique.

Of course, a new furrow is generated only when the landscape is ready for it. This would account for the fact that very often, whenever the ground is ready for a new discovery, several people will make this discovery at the same time.*

Conversely, whenever an area of the morphogenetic field does not flow, it becomes locally stagnant, and sediment accumulates. Thus, valleys are filled up, riverbeds disappear, and information is buried because of not being used.

The concept of morphogenetic field is an excellent tool to describe all the processes of evolution, whether evolution of the universe, evolution of species, cultural evolution, or personal evolution. It helps us understand how patterns are created.

On a personal level, one can see how positive thinking, for instance, can affect one's life, attracting positive experiences. This is why I am an incurable optimist, and why I think that pessimists are always wrong, especially when they are right.

Botanical families can be viewed as deep valleys in the vegetal morphogenetic field, dividing into the rivers of species and the streams of subspecies or chemotypes. Each of these valleys, rivers, and streams has been generated throughout the ages in close interaction with the local and global environment (other families and species, and the ecosystems supporting them, including microorganisms, animals, and humans).

We can see how the concept of morphogenetic field is in total agreement with the Gaia hypothesis. Our planet is a living organism. Humanity has brought consciousness to this organism—for a purpose, undoubtedly. This purpose cannot be the destruction of the planet. As conscious cells of this organism, we have a responsibility to take care of our planet. Otherwise, we behave like a virus in a sick body, and the organism will try to get rid of us. A lose—lose situation.

Our planet, the body we live in, is presently going through an acute toxic crisis. For those of you familiar with natural healing, this means that our planet will most probably need to go through a dramatic discharge process. But there is an emergency. No economic or other consideration can prevail against this absolute necessity. There is now an enormous worldwide awareness of this crisis. This can be viewed as a natural defense mechanism of our

---

*Interestingly enough, in the late 1970s, my research in logic and the theory of information came very close to the ideas that Rupert Sheldrake was developing (I talked about field of forms; he talks about morphogenetic fields). I presented a paper at the University of California at Berkeley in 1980 to explain my theories. I was not aware of Sheldrake at that time, nor was he aware of my work.

planet. We must capitalize on this movement and start acting now. We can do it, individually and collectively.

BACK TO THE BOTANICAL FAMILIES

Botanical Families and the Gaia Hypothesis

The vegetable kingdom appeared on our planet long before the animal kingdom. Through evolution, from the primitive moss or fern, it gradually differentiated to generate the thousands of species that we now know. This evolution was at first independent of the animal kingdom (but maybe it was preparing the ground for it—by producing oxygen, for instance). Then, when the first animals appeared on our planet (and they appeared because the morphogenetic field was ready for them), the two realms evolved in close interaction. For example, more and more vegetable species came to depend on insects for pollination. And of course, animals were totally dependent on plants for their subsistence.

It is not unreasonable to think that this interaction went very far; plants were not only food for the animal kingdom but were also medicine. Animals provided fertilizers; they carried the seeds and buried them, moved the ground with their feet, trimmed the bushes. If the Gaia hypothesis is well founded—and I believe it is—if our planet be viewed as a living organism, this is not surprising.

Certain plants became specialized in their interaction with the animal kingdom. Human intervention further accentuated this process; the plants that are now cultivated domestically have been "created" through a long selection process. The varieties of corn, wheat, apples, or potatoes that we buy in our supermarkets do not exist in the wild—they were produced through genetic breeding.

The study of botanical families, by going from the global (the vegetable kingdom) to the particular (the species and subspecies) through the differentiation process (the botanical families), gives us a better understanding of and appreciation for our living planet. Each plant has accumulated through the millions of years of its history the living memory of the vegetable kingdom, the memory of its family, the memory of its genus, of its species. All this information is here for us to share and respect. This is an ongoing miracle.

The Plant's Domain of Creativity

When we look at a plant from the perspective of the botanical family, we can learn a lot from the family itself. We also can learn from the part of the plant where its creativity is the most developed, and in studying aromatherapy, where its essential oil is produced.

Each family seems to have a privileged

domain of creativity. The Labiatae and Myrtacea produce their essential oils mostly in the leaves, while the rose produces them in the flower; the citruses in the flower, the fruit, and the leaves; the burseraceae in their exudate, and so on.

Evolution: Involution

Each plant goes from the physical sphere, with its germ and then the roots, through the vital sphere with the leaves and to the astral sphere with the flower in a natural evolution process. It then creates its fruit or seed in an involution back to the physical world.

Essential oils produced in the roots (angelica, vetiver) tend to have a very grounding energy; they have a foodlike quality to them. They are not very refined, but they usually are potent stimulants of the vital functions (especially digestion) of the organism. Typically, they are recommended for anemia.

The plant's leaf system corresponds to its vital body. Essential oils produced in the leaves (eucalyptus, niaouli, peppermint, etc.) have a strong affinity with the prajna energy, the respiratory system. They tone the vital body. Excessive development of the leaf system of a plant is a sign of etheric imbalance that can produce toxicity (as in some Umbelliferae).

The flower is the plant's ultimate achievement. Only the most spiritually evolved plants (such as the rose) can fully create at this level. The production of fragrance is then a sign of intense astral activity. Although the essential oils are found in extremely small amounts in the flowers, their fragrances are typically very intense, though refined in nature. The plants with the most intense floral creativity rarely produce any significant fruit or seed. These plants' creativity is exhausted there, and their creation does not belong to the physical plane any longer. Such fragrances have a tendency to be exhilarating (jasmine) or even intoxicating (narcissus).

The essential oils of flowers are then usually very refined and subtle but very hard to extract. They often are too far removed from the physical sphere to be extracted through steam distillation. (Neroli and rose are an exception, as they are particularly well-balanced plants; they both produce edible fruits: oranges and rose hips.) Very sensitive to temperature, their molecules break apart when exposed to heat. Some of them can be extracted by solvents (jasmine, tuberose, narcissus).

The oils produced in the seed bring us back fully into the physical world, being less sophisticated, more humble, and straightforward (citrus fruits, anise, fennel, coriander). They are invigorating and fortifying, and show a strong affinity with the digestive system (especially those seeds that are food or spices).

Trees and bushes also have the ability to create oils in their wood (sandalwood, cedarwood). Such oils are centering and equilibrating. Here the creative process is drawn into the heart of the wood. These oils have the power to open our consciousness to higher spheres without our losing control. They are particularly suited to rituals, meditation, and yoga.

Finally, many trees and bushes (myrrh, frankincense, conifers, cistus) produce odorous resins or gums. The essential oil then has a strong affinity for the glandular system. They control secretions, and show cosmetic and healing properties (skin care, wounds, ulcers).

SEVEN

Essential Oils in Botanical Families

BIRCH (*Betula lenta* and *Betula nigra;* Betulaceae)

Traditionally produced in northeastern United States.

Distillation of the bark; the oil is clear to yellowish.

Fragrance: balsamic, sweet, warm.

Used in liniments and unguents for muscular and articular aches.

Birch oil contains up to 98% methyl salicylate; therefore, this oil is quite often adulterated with the latter product. Two varieties of birch oil have been differentiated: northern birch oils, produced in Pennsylvania, Vermont, and New Hampshire (apparently this oil is no longer produced), and southern birch oil, produced in the southern part of the Appalachian mountains.

Wintergreen oil is similar to birch oil in its composition; however, it is no longer produced. Therefore, everything sold as wintergreen is either methyl salicylate or birch oil.

Organs: Kidneys, joints.

Medicinal Properties:
Diuretic.
Analgesic.
Purifying, drainer (lymphatic), cleanser.

Indications:
Rheumatism, arthritis, muscular and articular pains (one of the best remedies). Kidney and urinary tract disorders (cystitis, stones, mucous discharge, dropsy). Autointoxication caused by poor elimination of urea, cholesterol, glucose. Skin diseases.

BURSERACEAE (Dry Fire)

Essential Oils of the Family: Elemi, frankincense, myrrh.

Burseraceae grow in desert tropical areas where the intense cosmic activity promotes the formation of gum and etheric oils. Boswellia (myrrh, frankincense), the most characteristic representatives of the type, grow in the Arabian peninsula, in the most extreme climate of the planet. They are surrounded by a thin cloud of essential oils, which filters the sun's rays and freshens the air around them—hence their strong antiinflammatory action. Burseraceae act against inner fire in the body (bronchitis, cough, pleurisy, phthisis, consumption).

The gum oozes from incisions or natural fissures in the bark or the wood. It is cicatrizant, vulnerary, and has powerful healing properties. It is especially useful in diseases related to secretion (inflammation of the breast or the uterus).

Putrefaction cannot take place in the desert; the air is too dry, the fire too intense. Burseraceae condense the desert energy and therefore have strong antiputrescent strong effects on corpses. They have a salutary action on ulcers, gangrene, and gastric and intestinal fermentation.

The desert is also the place where the one who wants to go beyond the mundane and the superfluous finds an austere but powerful environ. There, everything is reduced to essentials. The contemplation of the endless petrified waves of the sandy dunes inspires one to go beyond the always-changing waves of one's own mind and connect with bare infinity and eternity. The powerful comforting scent of myrrh or frankincense carried by the burning wind of the desert gently soothes one's deepest wounds and gives one further inspiration in meditation.

Since antiquity, myrrh and frankincense have been extensively used as incense in rituals and religious ceremonies. They have a very pronounced soothing, comforting, fortifying, and elevating action on the soul and the spirit.

Type of Action: Cooling, drying, fortifying.

Domain of Action: Skin, lungs, secretion, mind, psychic centers.

Indications: Inflammations (skin, lungs, breast, uterus).

Elemi (*Canarium luzonicum*)

The gum is produced in the Philippines, Central America, and Brazil.

Distillation of the gum; the oil is colorless to slightly yellow.

Fragrance: pleasant, balsamic, resembling camphor, incense-like.

Used in perfumery and in some medical preparations.

Introduced in Europe in the fifteenth century, elemi was an ingredient in numerous balms, unguents, and liniments. It is still used in the balm of Fioraventi and other vulnerary preparations.

Medicinal Properties and Indications:

Similar to those of myrrh and frankincense.

Frankincense (*Boswellia carteri*)

The gum is produced in northeast Africa and southeast Arabia (Somalia, Ethiopia, Yemen); the supply has been quite erratic lately, because of the political confusion in these countries.

Distillation of the gum; the oil is clear or yellow.

Fragrance: characteristic (balsamic, camphor-like, spicy, woody, slightly lemony).

Used in cosmetics and perfumery; blends well with almost any scent; makes a good fixative.

One of the most highly priced substances of the ancient world, frankincense was once as valuable as gold. Its trade was one of the major economic activities in some Arabic countries, and its control provoked many local wars. The Queen of Sabah, a main producer of that time, undertook a perilous journey from Somalia to Israel and visited King Solomon to secure such a flourishing trade. Frankincense has been burned in temples since antiquity, especially by the Egyptians and the Hebrews; it is still used in the rites of some churches. Frankincense gum was traditionally used to fumigate sick persons and drive out the evil spirits causing the sickness. The Egyptians used it in their rejuvenating unguents.

Medicinal Properties and Indications:

Similar to those of myrrh.
Special action on breast inflammations and uterine disorders.

Pregnancy, birth preparation.

Myrrh (*Commiphora myrrha*)

The gum is produced in the same areas as frankincense, as well as Libya and Iran.

Distillation of the gum; the oil is yellow to reddish-brown, more or less fluid.

Fragrance: pleasant, balsamic, camphor-like, musty, incense-like.

Used in perfumery and cosmetics; blends well with many oils; makes a good fixative.

The history of myrrh is closely tied to that of frankincense. These two substances were among the precious drugs reserved for fumigations, embalming, unctions, and liturgical practices. The Egyptian papyrus, the Vedas, the Bible, and Koran mention the numerous uses of myrrh in ceremonies, in perfumery, and in medicine.

Myrrh was an ingredient of many unguents, elixirs, and other multipurpose antidotes.

Medicinal Properties:

Balsamic, expectorant.
Astringent, resolutive.
Antiinflammatory, antiseptic, antiputrescent, vulnerary, cicatrizant.
Affects mucous membrane.
Stimulant, tonic.
Sedative.

Indications:

Inflammations (breast, lungs, gangrene, infected wounds, ulcers).

Catarrhal conditions (head, lungs, stomach, intestines).
Tuberculosis, phthisis, bronchitis, cough.
Hemorrhages (uterine, pulmonary).
Pregnancy, childbirth.

CINNAMON (*Cinnamomum zeylanicum*; Lauraceae)

Produced in Ceylon (best quality), India, China.

Distillation of the bark; the oil is reddish-brown. The leaves are also distilled, but the quality of their oil is much lower.

Fragrance: characteristically spicy, burning.

Widely used in food industry, pharmacy, cosmetics, perfumery.

Certainly one of the oldest spices known, cinnamon was already the object of an important trade between India, China, and Egypt more than 4000 years ago. In 2700 B.C., the Chinese emperor Shen Nung called it "kwei" in his pharmacopeia. Cinnamon is often mentioned in the Bible; Yahveh ordered Moses to use it in the fabrication of the holy ointment. It was one of the most important drugs of the Greek and Roman pharmacopeia, and was quite renowned for its stomachic, diuretic, tonic, and antiseptic properties.

Medicinal Properties:
Stimulant (circulatory, cardiac, and pulmonary functions).
Antiseptic, antiputrescent.
Antispasmodic.
Aphrodisiac.
Parasiticide.
Irritant and convulsive in high doses.

Indications:
Flu, asthenia.
Spasms, intestinal infections.
Impotence.
Childbirth, labor (increase contractions).

CISTUS (*Cistus ladaniferus*; Cistaceae)

Produced in Spain, Cyprus.

Distillation of the branches: the oil is reddish-brown.

Fragrance: musky, balsamic.

Used in expensive perfumes: makes a good fixative; gives a natural musk note to the blends.

Cistus, or rock rose, is a small bush growing in dry rocky areas of the Mediterranean countries, especially in Crete and Cyprus. Its leaves naturally exude a gum called labdanum. This gum has been highly appreciated in perfumery, cosmetics, and medicine since antiquity and was one of the ingredients of the "holy ointment" of the Bible.

The gum sticks to the wool of sheep grazing on the hills as they walk through the bushes. Shepherds in Crete and Cyprus used to comb the wool of their sheep to collect the precious gum. Labdanum was also collected by whipping the bushes with a special whip, this method giving a much better quality. Unfortunately, both methods have now been abandoned, and labdanum is not produced any more.

Medicinal Properties:

Tonic, astringent.
Nervous sedative, antispasmodic.
Vulnerary.

Indications:

Diarrhea, dysentery, intestinal troubles.
Nervousness, insomnia.
Ulcers.

COMPOSITAE (Realization, Organization, Structure)

Essential Oils of the Family: Chamomile, everlasting, mugwort, tarragon.

Other oils of interest: arnica, calendula, tansy, yarrow, wormwood.

The compositae are characterized by their inflorescence, a collection of small flowers forming a unique superior entity. This basic simple structure is able to generate such a diversity that, with about 800 genera and 13,000 species, the compositae constitute the largest botanical family.

Unlike orchids, another large family with amazing floral variations, which are scarce and isolated, Compositae grow all over the world in large settlements. They live in almost every terrestrial zone, except the far north and the tropical forest, from seashores to mountain tops, from deserts to swamps, with a preference for open spaces widely exposed to light such as meadows and steppes.

Very adaptive, intensely related to light, Compositae live primarily in the floral sphere. Because they embody a perfect balance of etheric and astral forces, the therapeutic activity of the plants of this family shows great diversity.

Chamomile (*Anthemis nobilis, Anthemis mixta, Chamomilla matricaria, Ormenis multicolis*)

Produced in France, Morocco, Spain, Egypt.

Distillation of flowers; the oil of *Anthemis nobilis* (Roman chamomile) and *Anthemis mixta* is yellow, while the oil of *Chamomilla matricaria* is light blue and *Ormenis multicolis* (blue chamomile) is dark blue, owing to the presence of azulene.

Fragrance: refreshing, aromatic.

Used in perfumery, cosmetics, and pharmacy.

Dedicated to the sun by the Egyptians for its febrifuge properties, chamomile is probably one of the oldest known medicinal plants. It was regarded as the plant's physician and was thought to keep other plants in good health.

Interest in chamomile has recently been revived with the discovery of azulene, an excellent antiinflammatory agent, which is not present in the fresh flower but is formed when the plant is distilled.

Many different botanical species over the world are called chamomile. Roman chamomile (*Anthemis nobilis*) and German chamomile (*Chamomilla matricaria*) are the most commonly used in herbology. The oil called "Chamomile mixta" or "wild chamomile" is distilled from the wild in southern Spain and Morocco. Blue chamomile is distilled in Morocco and Egypt. A pineapple-scented chamomile grows throughout the United States. It has not been distilled as far as I know. Other varieties of chamomile grow in different parts of the world but are used only locally.

Roman chamomile is an excellent calming and soothing oil, and a good liver stimulant.

Matricaria (its German name means "mother herb") is especially indicated for female disorders.

See also the essential oil quick reference charts for the differences between the chamomiles.

Medicinal Properties:

Antiinflammatory (especially matricaria).
Antispasmodic, mild nervous sedative (children), anticonvulsive, antidepressant.
Emmenagogue.
Antianemic.
Febrifuge, sudorific.
Hepatic, cholagogue.
Antiseptic.
Analgesic.
Stimulant of leukocytosis.
Cicatrizant, vulnerary.
Local vasoconstrictor.

Indications:

Infectious diseases, fever.
Anemia.
Inflammation.
Migraine, depression, headache, convulsions, insomnia, vertigo, irritability, hysteria.
Dysmenorrhea, amenorrhea, vaginitis, menopausal problems, vulvar pruritus.
Liver and spleen congestion.
Painful digestion, digestive problems of children, gastralgia, gastritis.
Ulcers (stomach, intestines).
Colic, colitis.
Neuralgia, rheumatism.
Teething pains, toothache, gingivitis.
Earache.
Wounds, burns, boils, urticaria, dermatitis, skin diseases, skin care.
Conjunctivitis.
Pronounced effect on the mind and nervous system (anger, oversensitiveness, temper tantrums of children).

Matricaria is especially recommended for feminine diseases (painful or irregular period, excessive loss of blood, hemorrhage).

The whole plant is aerial, radiant; each beam terminates in a white and gold flower with a bulging receptacle, which encloses a drop of air. This flower manifests a subdued ardor, an appeased and soothing flame. Chamomile likes light; it grows on roadsides, open fields, light sandy soils. Its affinity for the air element and its particular connection with the aerial spheres indicate the strong therapeutic action of chamomile on the abnormal astral processes in the human organism. It is beneficent against spasms, convulsions, hypersensitivity, menstruation troubles, colic, and neuralgic aches.

Everlasting (*Helicrysum italicum*)

Produced in southern France, Italy, Yugoslavia.

Distillation of the whole plant; the oil is yellowish.

Fragrance: strongly aromatic.

Everlasting is a fairly new oil in aromatherapy. My friend Gilles Garcin, with whom I used to distill wild lavender in the southern Alps of France, might very well be the first one to have distilled the plant for aromatherapy (incidentally, he used Henri Viaud's distillery). It has proved to be valuable for wounds and bruises.

Medicinal Properties:

Antiinflammatory, antiphlogistic (according to Kurt Schnaubelt, it is even more potent than blue chamomile).
Cell regenerator.

Indications:

Hemorrhage.
Bruises, trauma.
Open wounds.

Mugwort (*Artemisia vulgaris, artemisia herba alba*)

Produced in Morocco and North Africa.

Distillation of the whole plant; the oil is yellowish-brown.

Fragrance: Strongly aromatic, slightly musky.

Named after the goddess Artemis (or Diana), protectress of virgins, mugwort had an ancient reputation as a specific for female cycles. It was also a magical plant, known to increase psychic power.

Organs: Female genitals.

Medicinal Properties:

Emmenagogue (abortive at high doses), regulator of the feminine cycle.
Antispasmodic.
Cholagogue, tonic, aperitive.
Vermifuge.

Indications:

Menstrual troubles (amenorrhea; dismenorrhea; scanty, insufficient, or excessive periods).
Hysteria, convulsion, epilepsy, nervous vomiting.
Ascariasis, oxyuriasis.

Tarragon (*Artemisia dracunculus*)

Produced in France, United States, Belgium.

The oil is obtained by distillation of the plant, almost colorless. The fragrance is anisey and aromatic.

Medicinal Properties:

Stimulant of the digestive system (stomach and intestine).
Antispasmodic.
Carminative, aperitive.
Vermifuge.

Indications:

Dyspepsia, hiccup.
Dystonia, weak digestion.
Aerophagy, fermentation.
Intestinal parasites.

CONIFERAE (The air element; light, inner warmth versus cold; verticality)

Essential Oils of the Family: Cedarwood, cypress, fir, juniper, pine, spruce thuja. Other oils of interest: cade, sabine, therebentine.

A wide belt of Coniferae circles around the frigid and temperate zones of both hemispheres, from the far north or far south and almost to the mountaintops, depending on altitude. In tropical zones they grow only at high altitudes.

The type is imposing in its simplicity. It is dominated by a vertical and linear principle. Everything is structured around the central vertical trunk; the trunk is surrounded with branches shaped like small trees, and the leaves are reduced to long needles placed in spirals around the twigs. The floral process is reduced to its minimum: the cone of flowers, a terminal twig surrounded by dense ligneous leaves, bears the nude reproductive organs (stamens or pistil) on the axil of its leaves.

The longevity of Coniferae, ruled by Saturn, gives us the oldest and highest trees in the world. In some species, the trunks themselves are virtually immune to rot (prehistoric cypresses found in coal mines in Silesia were used to make furniture!)

The coniferous forest appears immemorial and eternal. Its solemnity, its noble majesty, its powerful magnificence bring us back to primordial nature. This forest inspires devotion and respect and opens the heart "to the most ancient, the most basic and primordial feelings of the creation" (Goethe). Troubled souls find rest and strength there.

Coniferae also produce in abundance etheric oils and resins, which fill up the trunks, branches, and needles. In certain species, the resin production is so intense that the trees exude it through their cones or their trunks. Such a phenomenon indicates a deep characteristic relationship between this type and the forces of light and warmth. Because Coniferae live in cold climates, they have to develop an intense inner fire in order to face the long, rigorous winters until the overflowing light of summer, with its clear nights and its midnight sun. These processes of warmth relate to life and generate substances (essential oils, resins, balms) and are at the origin of the curative power of Coniferae, which is warming and revivifying. Their zone of action is the cold area of the body: the nervous system.

Type of Action: Tonic, revivifying, appeasing, warming.

Domain of Action: Nervous system, lungs, glandular system.

Indications:

Stress, deficiency of the nervous system.
Lung problems.
Rheumatism, arthritis.

The oils of Coniferae are best taken through the lungs (inhalation, aromatic diffuser), where they communicate the *prajna* of the type.

Cedarwood (*Cedrus atlantica*)

Produced in Morocco.

Cedrus deodorata is distilled in the Himalayas. The cedar of Virginia, distilled in the United States, is a juniper (*Juniperus virginiana* and *Juniperus mexicana*); the oil, however, is very close to real cedarwood oil.

Distillation of the sawdust; the oil is thick and golden-brown, like the color of old gold.

Fragrance: deep, woody, balsamic, very pleasant, like sandalwood.

Used as a fixative in perfumes; blends well with many oils and gives a woody note to preparations.

Egyptians used cedarwood oil for embalming; it was one of the ingredients of *mithridat*, a famous poison antidote that was used for centuries.

Medicinal Properties:

Antiseptic, fungicidal, antiputrescent.
Expectorant.
Stimulant.

Indications:

Cystitis, gonorrhea, urinary tract disorders.
Hair care (hair loss, dandruff, scalp diseases).
Respiratory conditions.
Skin diseases (eczema, dermatitis, ulcers).
Anxiety, nervous tension.

One of the most majestic trees, the Lebanese cedar (like its close relative, atlas cedar, growing in Morocco) expresses a great spiritual strength. Egyptians used its wood to build the doors of their temples, where its fragrance would stimulate psychic centers of the worshipers. The effects of cedarwood oil on the mind are similar to that of sandalwood.

Cypress (*Cupressus sempervirens*)

Produced in France, Spain, Morocco.

Distillation of branches; the oil is yellow to brown.

Fragrance: balsamic, woody, somewhat harsh.

The ancient Egyptians used cypress in their medical preparations; its wood, almost immune to rot, was used to make the sarcophagi for the mummies.

Medicinal Properties:

Astringent, vasoconstrictor, tonic for the veins.
Antispasmodic.
Diuretic, antirheumatic, antisudorific.
Antiseptic.

Indications:
   Hemorrhoids, varicose veins.
   Enuresis.
   Whooping cough, asthma.
   Ovary dysfunction (dysmenorrhoea, menopausal problems).
   Perspiration.

Fir (*Abies balsamea*)

Produced in northeast United States and Canada.
   Distillation of branches.
   Fragrance: fresh, balsamic, very pleasant; one of the finest coniferous scents.

   The fir pine tree exudes a resin called fir balsam that the North American Indians used for medicinal and religious purposes. It was introduced in Europe in the beginning of the seventeenth century, and its action was compared to that of Venetian turpentine, highly valued at the time.

Medicinal Properties:
   Respiratory antiseptic, expectorant.
   Vulnerary.

Indications:
   Respiratory diseases.
   Genitourinary infections.

Juniper (*Juniperus communis*)

Produced in Yugoslavia, Italy, and France.
   Distillation of the berries (gives the best quality) or the small branches; the oil is colorless, yellowish, or pale green.
   Fragrance: terebenthinate, hot, balsamic.
   Juniper was burned as incense, to ward off evil spirits or to serve as a disinfectant in time of epidemic diseases. Tibetans used it for religious and medicinal purposes.

Medicinal Properties:
   Diuretic, antiseptic (urinary tract), anti-rheumatic (promotes the elimination of uric acid and toxins).
   Stomachic.
   Antidiabetic.
   Tonic: nervous system, visceral functions, digestive system.
   Fortifies the memory.
   Rubefacient.
   Vulnerary.

Indications:
   Urinary tract infections, kidney stones, blennorrhoea, cystitis, oliguria.
   Diabetes.
   Rheumatism, arteriosclerosis.
   General weariness, nervous fatigue.
   Amenorrhea, dysmenorrhea, painful menstruation.
   Dermatitis, eczema.

The smallest of coniferae grows in arid and inhospitable areas, where its presence is like a consolation. During Christmas ceremonies in Germany, it represents the tree of life. It hides its rough, bitter fruits in the midst of thick needles; these fruits are salutary for everyone who has abused terrestrial food. It is an excellent diuretic, digestive, and hepatic.

Its distorted shape and hard, knotty, twisted wood indicate an obvious affinity with joints, arthritis, and rheumatism. Juniper can deal with the diseases of old age.

Pine (*Pinus sylvestris*)

Produced in the U.S.S.R., Germany, and France, *Pinus maritimus* is distilled in France. Various species closely related to *Pinus sylvestris* are distilled in Austria, Italy, and Yugoslavia.

Distillation of small branches; the oil is colorless.

Medicinal Properties:
Expectorant, pulmonary antiseptic.
Stimulant of adrenocortical glands.
Hepatic and urinary antiseptic.
Rubefacient.

Indications:
Pulmonary diseases.
Urinary infections.

Spruce (*Picea mariana*)

Produced in the same area as fir.
Distillation of branches; the oil is colorless.
Fragrance: similar to fir, but deeper.

Medicinal Properties and Indications:
Same as fir.

Spruce oil is excellent for balancing the energy. It is recommended for any type of psychic work for its opening and elevating, though grounding, quality. In the diffuser, it is excellent for yoga and meditation.

Thuja (*Thuja occidentalis*)

Produced in Canada, United States (Vermont, New Hampshire).

The oil is obtained by distillation of small branches and twigs and has a yellowish color. It is highly toxic and therefore should not be taken internally without the supervision of a medical specialist.

Medicinal Properties:
Diuretic, urinary sedative.
Expectorant.
Antirheumatic.
Vermifuge.

Indications:
Prostatic hypertrophy, cystitis.
Rheumatism.
Intestinal parasites.
Warts.

GERANIUM (*Pelargonium graveolens & roseum*; Geraniaceae)

Produced in Reunion, Comoro Islands, Egypt, Morocco.

Distillation of the plant; the oil is greenish-yellow.

Fragrance: strong, sweet, roselike (almost too strong when it is pure but becomes very pleasant when diluted).

Widely used in perfumery and cosmetics; blends very well with rose, citrus, and almost any oil.

Old herbals mention geranium or Herb-Robert (*Geranium robertianum*), which grows wild in the temperate zones of the globe. This plant is totally different from the pelargonium used for the extraction of essential oils. Although they both belong to the same botanical family, their uses are different.

It has been recently discovered that geranium has the power to develop an extremely wide variety of chemotypes, none of them being distilled commercially at this point. The reasons for such variations are not yet clear.

In fact, geranium can be made to imitate almost any fragrance. Besides the rose geranium, tangerine geranium, lemon geranium, lime geranium, etc. are found in nurseries. Apparently, the species can produce almost any possible chemotype, including the hot, burning thymols and carvacrols that seem so remote from the sweet-smelling rose geranium that most people know. This seems to indicate a strong adaptability, indicative of immunostimulant properties.

Organs: Kidneys.

Medicinal Properties:
Astringent, hemostatic, cicatrizant, antiseptic.

Antidiabetic, diuretic.
Stimulant of adrenal cortex.
Insect repellent.

Indications:
Diabetes, kidney stones.
Adrenocortical deficiency.
Tonsillitis, sore throat.
Hemorrhage.
Burns, wounds, ulcers.
Skin diseases, skin care.
Nervous tension, depression.

GINGER (*Zingiber officinale*; Zingiberaceae)

Produced in China, India, Malaysia.

Distillation of the rhizome; the oil is slightly yellow to dark yellow.

Fragrance: characteristic (camphor-like, aromatic, citrusy).

Widely used in the eastern countries (especially India, China, Japan) in pharmaceutical preparations. Many uses in the food and beverage industries.

Ginger has been used for thousands of years in India and China for its remarkable medicinal properties and for its culinary uses. It is still one of the major remedies prescribed by macrobiotic therapists and Chinese doctors. Dioscorides recommends it for digestion and stomach weakness. It was mentioned in the Middle Ages as a tonic, stimulant, and febrifuge. It is an ingredient of the balm of Fioraventi.

Organs: Digestive system.

Medicinal Properties:
  Tonic, stimulant.
  Stomachic, carminative.
  Analgesic.
  Febrifuge.
  Antiscorbutic.

Indications:
  Deficiency of the digestive system (dyspepsia, flatulence, loss of appetite, etc.).
  Impotence.
  Rheumatic pain.

GRAMINAE (The Nutritious Family)

Essential Oils of the Family: Citronella, lemongrass, litsea cubeba, palmarosa, vetiver.

A wide majority of the plants covering the ground belong to the Graminae family. From the poles to the equator, from the swamps to the deserts, this family shows an amazing adaptability and diversity. Its ability to cover almost exclusively huge areas denotes a singular strength. This strength lies in the powerful root system, forming an intricate network that blends almost perfectly with the soil (modern gardeners, in order to create lawns, lay on the soil a kind of carpet which is vegetal and ground together). Above this intense root system, the aerial part of Graminae is dominated by a linear principle: long narrow leaves and straight stems. Even the inflorescence (ear) obeys this principle.

The family does not spend much energy in the floral process — it is entirely dedicated to another aim: Graminae above all is the nutritious family. Its leaves and seeds are a present to the animal kingdom: grass for herbivores, grain (wheat, rice, corn, barley, oats) for rodents, birds, and humans.

The family has the potential to develop fragrances. Just remember the scent of freshly cut hay! But it usually remains a potential, a nascent fragrance. Only under the tropics has this ability been fully developed in some species. The herbs of lemongrass, citronella litsea cubeba, and palmarosa have a fresh, green, lemony, slightly rosy fragrance. Vetiver produces essential oils in its roots.

Citronella (*Cymbopogon nardus*)

Produced in China, Malaysia, Sri Lanka, Central America.
  Distillation of the herb; the oil is yellow.
  Fragrance: fresh, green, lemony.
  Widely used in the soap industry, deodorizers, insecticide, sanitary products. Few uses in perfumery. The herb is used in Chinese food.

Medicinal Properties and Indications:
  Disinfection of rooms, insecticide.

Lemongrass (*Cymbopogon citratus*)

Produced in India, Central America, and Brazil. *Cymbopogon flexuosus* produces an essential oil also called Indian verbena (not the real essential oil of verbena, which is 10 times more expensive).

Distillation of the herb: the oil is yellow to reddish-brown.

Fragrance: fresh, lemony, finer than citronella.

Widely used in the soap industry and in perfumery. Veterinary uses: parasites, digestive troubles.

According to the Indian pharmacopeia, lemongrass was traditionally used by the Indian as an antidote against infectious diseases, fevers, and cholera.

Medicinal Properties:
Stimulant of the digestive system (stomachic, carminative, digestive).
Antiseptic.
Diuretic.
Insect repellent.

Indications:
Digestive troubles (dyspepsia, colic, flatulence).
Disinfection, deodorization.
Pediculosis, scabies.

Litsea cubeba

Produced in China.
Distillation of the herb; the oil is yellow.
Fragrance: fresh, green, lemony.
Widely used in perfumery and in the soap industry, deodorizers, sanitary products.

Although it is closely related to citronella and lemongrass, Litsea cubeba has a much nicer fragrance. It is a fairly new oil in aromatherapy, mostly used for blending (especially in the diffuser). It gives a pleasant fresh, lemony top note to any blend.

Medicinal Properties and Indications:
Same as lemongrass.

Palmarosa (*Cymbopogon martini*)

Produced in India, Africa, Comoro Islands, Madagascar.
Distillation of the herb; the oil is yellow.
Fragrance: fresh, rose-like.
Widely used in perfumery and cosmetology (and to adulterate rose oil, one of the most expensive essential oils).

Medicinal Properties:
Antiseptic cellular stimulant, hydrating.
Febrifuge.
Digestive stimulant.

Indications:
Skin care: wrinkles, acne, etc. (reestablishes the physiological balance of the skin, immediate calming and refreshing action).
Digestive atonia.

Vetiver (*Andropogon muricatus*)

Produced in Comoro Islands, Caribbean islands, Reunion.
The oil is obtained from the roots; it is deep brown and very thick.

Fragrance: deep, hearty, woody (slightly reminiscent of tobacco plant or clary), musky, sandalwood-like.

Used mostly in perfumery and cosmetics; makes a very good fixative.

Indication: Arthritis.

With vetiver, the aromatic process is drawn into the roots, wherein lies the power of Graminae. Its fragrance is then an actualization in the odoriferous sphere of the potentialities that the type usually expresses in the nutritious sphere. The characteristic earthy, realistic, almost materialistic scent definitively accounts for the nutritious aspect of the family, while the musky note reminds one of its animal connection.

Graminae produce the most sacred food of the vegetable kingdom: wheat, rice, and corn—food beyond food, gift of the gods to the human realm. Vetiver expresses this fundamental aspect of the type through its sandalwood-like note; it is inspiring and uplifting.

JASMINE (*Jasminum officinalis*)

Produced in southern France, North Africa (Egypt, Tunisia, Morocco), and India.

There is no essential oil of jasmine. The oil is obtained by either enfleurage or solvent extraction (see Chapter III). In enfleurage, fresh flowers are placed on top of a blend of fats (usually a mixture of pork fat, beef fat, and vegetable oils). The fat absorbs the fragrance released by the flower. The old flowers are removed every day and fresh flowers are placed on the fat. This process yields a product called pomade. The pomade is then washed with alcohol to remove the fats; next, the alcohol is removed through vacuum distillation to produce the absolute from enfleurage.

Enfleurage is very time-consuming and has generally been abandoned; only a few producers are still using this process. Nowadays, natural fats are replaced by a solvent (hexane, a petroleum derivative). The products obtained are called concrete (usually waxy) and absolute.

Jasmine absolute is brown and rather viscous.

Fragrance: deep, sweet, warming, long-lasting, exhilarating, supremely exotic.

Blends beautifully with rose, neroli, bergamot, petitgrain, sandalwood, citruses, palmarosa, geranium, rosewood.

With rose and neroli, jasmine is one of the major "noble" oils of perfumery. It is also one of the most expensive oils; therefore it is very often adulterated.

Medicinal Properties:
 Aphrodisiac, stimulant of sexual chakra.
 Antidepressant.
 Childbirth preparation.

Indications:
 Impotence, frigidity.
 Anxiety, depression, lethargy, lack of confidence.
 Postnatal depression.
 Makes a fine perfume.

If rose is the oil of love, jasmine is certainly the oil of romance and was revered as such in the Hindu and Muslim traditions. It inspired burning lascivious songs to the Arab poets. In the harem, the prince's favorite soaked in a jasmine-scented bath and received an elaborate jasmine massage to induce sensual ecstasy in her lover.

Supremely sensual, jasmine is certainly the best aphrodisiac that aromatherapy can offer. It should not be considered a mere sexual stimulant, though. Jasmine releases inhibition, liberates imagination, and develops exhilarating playfulness. In a way, the power of jasmine can only be fully experienced by real lovers, as it has the power to transcend physical love and fully release both male and female sexual energy. It is the best stimulant of the sexual chakra and is recommended for any type of kundalini work.

LABIATAE (Plants of Heat)

Essential Oils of the Family: Basil, clary sage (see *Salvia*), hyssop, lavender, lavandin (see lavender), marjoram, melissa, oregano, patchouli, pennyroyal (see mints), peppermint (see mints), rosemary, sage (see *Salvia*), spearmint (see mints), spike (see lavender), thyme.

While medicinal plants are the exception in most families, all Labiatae have some curative power, which indicates their special relationship to humans. This phenomenon is due to the extraordinary influence of the cosmic forces of heat on the formation of the family. This calorific nature leads to the formation of essential oils.

Labiatae have a special predilection for open spaces; dry, rocky slopes; and sunny mountains, where their most characteristic species appear (lavender, rosemary, sage, thyme). They prefer median climatic regions: all around the Mediterranean, and far from tropical and cold areas.

Many Labiatae are culinary herbs, which indicates their affinity for the digestive processes. Their fragrance is invigorating, stimulating, fiery, reawakening. There are no bland, gloomy, ecstatic, or narcotic notes in this family.

Finally, many Labiatae (basil, peppermint, rosemary, thyme) have the power to develop chemotypes (see Chapter IV, The Chemistry of Common Essential Oil Constituents). This seem to indicate a strong potential for adaptability in the family, which could be interpreted as immunostimulant power. (Geranium is another plant with many chemotypes, and it is also considered an immunostimulant.)

Type of Action:
Warming, stimulating (vital center, metabolism).

Appeasing effect on overactive astral body; brings it back under the control of vital centers.

Domain of Action:
Organization of vital centers:

Metabolism, digestion, respiration, blood formation.

Indications:
Weakness of vital centers (anemia, poor digestion, respiratory problems, diabetes).
Recommended for people with intense psychic activity (healers, mediums, etc.) to keep them from losing control and depleting their vitality.

Basil (*Ocymum basilicum*)

Produced in India, Egypt, Comoro Islands, Reunion.
Distillation of the herb; the oil is yellow.
Fragrance: Pleasant, anisey, with a minty note.
Used in perfumery for its top green note; blends well with bergamot or geranium.
There are several chemotypes of basil (there is even a cinnamon basil); the most commonly used in the methylchavicol type (Reunion and Comoro Islands), the eugenol type also being used.
One of the sacred plants of India, where it is dedicated to Vishnu, basil is extensively used in Ayurvedic medicine. Its actions on the digestive and nervous systems have been acknowledged in both Indian and occidental medicine.

Organs: Neurovegetative and digestive systems.

Medicinal Properties:
Nervous tonic, antispasmodic, cephalic.
Stomachic, intestinal antiseptic.
Stupefying at high doses.

Indications:
Mental fatigue, migraine, insomnia, depression, mental strain.
Dyspepsia, gastric spasms.
Intestinal infections.
Facilitates birth and nursing.

Hyssop (*Hyssopus officinalis*)

Produced in France, Spain, southern Europe.
Distillation of the whole plant in flower; the oil is golden-yellow.
Fragrance: nicely aromatic, reminiscent of sage, marjoram, and lavender.
One of the sacred plants of the Hebrews, hyssop (*esobh*) was prescribed by Hippocrates, Galen, and Dioscorides for its curative power on the respiratory system. The ancient pharmacopeia mention it as the major ingredient in numerous preparations, elixirs, and syrups.

Organs: Lungs.

Medicinal Properties:
Expectorant (liquify bronchial secretions), antitussive, emollient.
Antispasmodic.
Tonic (especially heart and respiration).
Hypertensive agent, regulates blood pressure.
Digestive, stomachic.
Sudorific, febrifuge.
Cicatrizant, vulnerary.

Indications:
Hypotension.

Respiratory diseases (asthma, bronchitis, catarrh, cough, tuberculosis).
Poor digestion, dyspepsia, flatulence.
Dermatitis, eczema, wounds.
Syphilis.
Urinary stones.

Hyssop grows all over southern Europe and western Asia on dry, rocky slopes, but its finest varieties grow above 3000 feet in the sunny meadows of the southern Alps. Its abundant leaf system and its camphor-like scent indicate its special affinity for the respiratory system.

Lavender (*Lavandula officinalis*)

One of the most precious essential oils.
Produced in France, Spain, U.S.S.R.
Distillation of flowers; the oil is clear, yellowish-green.
Fragrance: clean, classic, appeasing.
Best variety: "lavender fine"; others: Mayette, materonne.
Lavender was a favorite aromatic for use by the Romans in their baths (the word comes from the Latin *lavare*). Dioscorides, Pliny, and Galen mention it as a stimulant, tonic, stomachic, and carminative. It has always been used in perfumery and cosmetics and blends well with a great number of essential oils, adding a light floral note to almost any preparation.

Medicinal Properties:
Calming, analgesic, antispasmodic, anti-convulsive, antidepressant.
Antiseptic, healing.

Cytophylactic.
Diuretic, antirheumatic.
Insect repellent.

Indications:
Respiratory diseases (asthma, bonchitis, catarrh, influenza, whooping cough, throat infections).
Sinusitis.
Migraine, depression, convulsions, nervous tension, fainting, insomnia, neurasthenia, palpitations.
Infectious diseases.
Skin diseases: abscess, acne, dermatitis, eczema, pediculosis, psoriasis.
Burns, wounds.
Leukorrhea.
Cystitis, mucous discharge.
Insect bites.

Far from the ardor of rosemary, lavender emanates a noble, mellow peacefulness. Its blue flowers bloom at the top of a structure resembling a seven-branched candlestick; they give a clean, soothing scent that is one of our most beautiful perfumes.

The finest quality grows above 3000 feet on the sunny slopes of the southern Alps and up to the mountain top. Lavender likes air, space, light, and warmth. It has an appeasing action on the astral body; it tones and soothes the nervous system and is beneficial for the respiratory system.

Spike (*Lavendula spica*)

Spike grows below 2000 feet. Its essential oils contain some camphor; it calms the cerebrospinal activity. It is also used as an insecticide and for veterinary purposes.

Lavandin (*Lavandula fragrans, delphinensis*)

The lavandins are hybrids of true lavender and spike; their essential oils have a lower ester content and contain some camphor. Their fragrance is not as refined as that of lavender; their medicinal properties are similar, to a lesser degree.

Main varieties: super and abrialis (the finest), grosso.

Veterinary Uses: Antiseptic, vulnerary, dermatitis, scabies.

Marjoram (*Origanum marjorana, Marjorana hortensi*)

Other variety: wild spanish marjoram (*Thymus mastichina*).

Produced in Spain (wild Spanish marjoram), Egypt, North Africa, Hungary.

Distillation of the plant in flower.

Fragrance: sweet, appeasing, one of the nicest of Labiatae oils.

Used in perfumery and cosmetics; blends well with lavender and bergamot.

Marjoram was grown in ancient Egypt. Greeks and Romans used it to weave crowns for the newly married. According to mythology, Aphrodite, goddess of love and fecundity, picked marjoram on Mount Ida to heal the wounds of Enea. According to Dioscorides, it tones and warms the nerves;

Pliny recommends it for poor digestion and a weak stomach; Culpepper praises its warming and comforting effects.

Organs: Peripheral nervous system.

Medicinal Properties:
Antispasmodic, calming, sedative, analgesic, anaphrodisiac.
Hypotensor, arterial vasodilator.
Digestive.
Narcotic in high doses.

Indications:
Spasms (digestive, pulmonary), insomnia, migraine, nervous tension, neurasthenia, anxiety.
Hypertension.
Dyspepsia, flatulence.
Arthritis, rheumatic pain.

Rather than altitude and rocks, marjoram prefers the light warm soil of gardens. The plant is sweet-looking and delicate, with small, round, soft, velvety leaves and cute little white flowers, almost hidden among the leaves. Its gentle and appeasing fragrance has a warming and comforting effect, hence its beneficent action on the nervous system. Marjoram also has a warming action on the metabolism and genital organs.

Melissa (*Melissa officinalis*)

Produced in France.
Distillation of the plant.
Fragrance: fresh, lemony, very pleasant.

Melissa (sometimes called balm or lemon balm, or *citronelle* in French) has a very low yield (about 0.05%). The production of the oil had been virtually abandoned until the late 1980s when a few French producers started distilling it again. It is a very expensive oil, and is therefore widely adulterated (most common adulterations are lemongrass, citronella, and litsea cubeba). So-called melissa oil has been offered (even when it was not produced), especially in England, at a fraction of the production cost of true melissa oil. While total world production of melissa oil was less than 50 pounds in 1988, total sales worldwide could have been well over 1000 pounds. Another miracle of modern technology!

Patricia Davis, in her excellent *Aromatherapy: An A–Z*, warns against possible skin irritations when using melissa oil externally. One wonders whether she used true melissa oil in the first place, since most of what is available for purchase is adulterated.

Medicinal Properties:
Antispasmodic, calming, sedative, soothing.
Antidepressant, uplifing.
Digestive.
Antivirus.
Stimulant of the heart chakra.

Indications:
Insomnia.
Migraine, nervous tension, neurasthenia, anxiety.
Cold sores, shingles.
Emotional shock, grief.

The plant is named after the Greek nymph Melissa, protectress of the bees. In spring, when several queens are born in the same beehive, the swarm splits into several smaller swarms, and each has to look for a new hive. Fresh leaves were traditionally crushed on empty hives to attract the migrant swarms.

Melissa is a gentle and humble-looking plant with pale green leaves and small white flowers. There emanates from the whole plant a natural kindness that is soothing and comforting in itself. Melissa was traditionally considered calming and uplifting. It is very soothing, relieves tension, and is, with rose and neroli, one of the major oils of the heart chakra.

Melissa seems to thrive on iron. It likes the vicinity of houses, especially in the country (nails and other pieces of scrap iron are often buried around habitations). When I was a wildcrafter, the place where I could find the most abundant crop of melissa was an abandoned iron mine.

This indicates a possible antianemic and immunostimulant property; melissa has been known to strengthen vitality.

Mints (Pennyroyal, Peppermint, Spearmint)

Pluto once fell in love with the nymph Mintha, but his wife, the jealous Proserpine, changed her into the plant that is now named after her. According to Pliny, "The scent of mint awakens the mind and its taste excites the appetite and the stomach." Its fortifying and stimulating qualities have been acknowledged by Roman and Greek physicians.

There are about 20 species in the genus *Mentha*, growing all over the world. They like abundant light and deep, humid soils. In them, the warmth principle struggles against an adverse principle of cold and water, hence there is a warming, stimulating, curative power, good to resolve congestion, cramps, and swelling, and to promote menstruation and virility. On the other hand, mints also have vivifying, refreshing, and appeasing qualities.

Common Medicinal Properties of the Genus *Mentha:*

Stimulant of nervous system, general, tonic, antispasmodic.
Stomachic, digestive, carminative.
Hepatic, cholagogue.
Expectorant.
Emmenagogue.
Febrifuge.
Antiseptic.

Indications:

Gastralgia, dyspepsia, nausea, flatulence, vomiting.
Mental fatigue, migraine, headache, fainting, neuralgia.
Dysmenorrhea.
Hepatic disorders.
Cold, cough, asthma, bronchitis.
Neuralgia.

Pennyroyal (*Mentha pelugium*)

Produced in Spain, North Africa.
Distillation of the plant.
Fragrance: resembling peppermint, but harsher.

Specific Medicinal Properties and Indications:

Amenorrhea (warning: pennyroyal is abortive at high doses)
Splenetic

Peppermint (*Mentha piperita*)

Produced all over the world, the United States being the biggest producer; the finest quality comes from England and southern France.
Distillation of the plant.
Numerous uses in perfumery, cosmetics, and food industry (liquors, sauces, drinks, candies, etc.).
Mentha piperita has several subspecies and chemotypes (*Mentha piperita* var. *bergamia*, or chemotype linalol, etc.), none of them being commercially distilled as far as I know.

Specific Indications: Impotence.

Spearmint (*Mentha viridis*)

The fragrance of spearmint is very similar to that of peppermint, but is fresher and less harsh. Its therapeutic activity is approximately the same.

Oregano (*Origanum vulgare, Origanum compactum, Corido-thymus capitatus*)

Produced in Spain, North Africa, Greece (many subspecies).

Distillation of the herb; the oil is brownish-red.

Fragrance: burning, spicy, strongly aromatic.

Although the ancients often grouped different species under this name, oregano had been considered an essential aromatic plant for medicine and for cooking since antiquity. Theophrastes, Aristotle, and Hippocrates praised its beneficent action on respiratory diseases, ulcers, burns, and poor digestion.

Medicinal Properties:

Antiseptic, antitoxic, antivirus.
Antispasmodic, sedative.
Expectorant.
Analgesic, counterirritant.

Indications:

Infectious diseases, disinfection.
Bronchopulmonary diseases.
Rheumatism.
Pediculosis.
Amenorrhea.

A rustic variant of marjoram, oregano grows wild all over Europe and Asia; however, only the Mediterranean varieties yield a significant amount of essential oils. Their hot, almost burning quality indicates their beneficent action on infectious diseases, infected wounds, and inflammations.

Patchouli (*Pogostemon patchouli*)

Produced in India, Malaysia, Burma, Paraguay.

The leaves are dried and fermented prior to distillation; the oil is thick, brown to greenish-brown.

Fragrance: strong, sweet, musty, very persistent.

Used in dermatology, aesthetics, and skin care. One of the best fixatives, used in small amounts in oriental and rose perfumes.

Patchouli essential oil was part of the *materia medica* in Malaysia, China, India, and Japan, where it was used for its stimulant, tonic, stomachic, and febrifuge properties. It was a renowned antidote against insect and snake bites.

The Indians also used it to scent their fabrics, especially the famous Indian shawls so fashionable in England in the nineteenth century.

The oil contains patchoulene and other products close to azulene.

Medicinal Properties:

Decongestive, antiphlogistic, antiinflammatory, tissue regenerator.
Fungicide, antiinfectious, bactericide.
Stimulant (nervous system) at low doses.
Sedative at high doses.
Rejuvenating to the skin.
Insect repellent.

Indications:

Mucous discharge, sluggishness; skin care (seborrhea, eczema, dermatitis, impetigo, herpes, cracked skin, wrinkles).
Anxiety, depression.
Insect and snake bites.

One of the most tropical Labiatae, patchouli is a plant of excessive warmth and water; however, its large leaves and its morphology indicate that these energies are not fully dominated. Therefore, though it is stimulant and tonic at low doses, good for dissipating the type of lethargy related to such energies (sluggishness, inertia), it become sedative or even stupefying at high doses. Its antiinflammatory and decongestive properties also derive from these characteristics.

Because the oil is produced after a period of fermentation, it has a certain control on all processes of stagnation, putrefaction, and aging (uses in skin care, rejuvenation). *Opus niger* (black work), which in the physical world is a process of fermentation and putrefaction, is one of the major phases of the alchemist's work, a phase conducive to the illumination of the adept after cold burning of all impurities and decantation. Patchouli is then a product of fermentation in the alchemical sense. It has a powerful action on the psychic centers on a metaphysical level.

Rosemary (*Rosmarinus officinalis*)

Produced all around the Mediterranean sea.

Distillation of herb; oil almost colorless.

Fragrance: fiery, aromatic, invigorating, with a dominant note reminiscent of eucalyptus (for the Spanish and North African varieties), and reminiscent of frankincense (more pronounced in the French or Yugoslavian varieties).

Like thyme, but to a lesser degree, Rosemary has developed several chemotypes, growing in fairly distinct climatic areas. The phenol-cineol chemotype grows in North Africa (Morocco, Tunisia), the cineol chemotype grows in Spain, and the verbenon chemotype grows in southern France, Corsica, northern Italy, and Yugoslavia.

This vigorous, thick bush with a predilection for rocky, sunny slopes grows all around the Mediterranean, from the seashore to about 2000 feet. It has been extensively used since antiquity for medicine and in cooking as well as for rituals.

Highly praised in the Middle Ages and the Renaissance, it appeared in various formulas such as the famous "water of the Queen of Hungary," a rejuvenating liquor. Elizabeth of Hungary received the recipe from an angel (or a monk) at the age of 72, gouty and paralytic. She recovered health and beauty, and the King of Poland even wanted to marry her!

Madame de Sevigny recommended rosemary water for sadness.

Organs: Liver, gallbladder.

Medicinal Properties:

General stimulant, cardiotonic, stimulant of adrenocortical glands.

Cholagogue, hepatobiliary stimulant (increases biliary secretion).

Pulmonary antiseptic.

Diuretic, sudorific.

Antirheumatismal, antineuralgic, rubefacient.

Healing of wounds and burns.

Indications:

Hepatobiliary disorders (cholecystitis, cirrhosis, gallstones, hypercholesterolaemia, jaundice).

General weakness, anemia, asthenia, debility, menstruation.

Mental fatigue, mental strain, loss of memory.

Colds, bronchitis, whooping cough.

Rheumatism, gout.

Hair loss, dandruff.

Skin care.

Wounds, burns.

Scabies, pediculosis.

A calorific plant above all, according to Rudolf Steiner rosemary fortifies the vital center and its action of the other constituents of the human being. It restores the balance of the calorific body and activates the blood processes (blood is the privileged medium of the heating principle in the human body). It is thus recommended for anemia, insufficient menstruation, and troubles of blood irrigation. It acts on the liver as well.

A better irrigation of the organs eases the action of astral and viral forces and stimulates metabolism: rosemary is digestive and sudorific; it promotes the assimilation of sugar (in diabetes) and is indicated to rebuild the nervous system after long, intense intellectual activity.

The Genus *Salvia*

With over 500 species, the genus *Salvia* is the most important of the Labiatae family.

Salvia officinalis likes chalky rocks and the desert mountains of Spain, Greece, Dalmatia, and the Balkans. Its fragrance is severe, solemn, earthy, and harsh. Its well-developed leaves, and large odoriferous flowers shaped to receive the bodies of bees, indicate its affinity for all processes of life and creation—even procreation. *Salvia sclarea* goes even further; reduced for years to a few small leaves close to the ground, it suddenly develops wide, thick leaves and extravagant flowers atop high, square stems, suggesting the quiet confidence and radiance of a pregnant woman. It was preeminently the plant of women in their creative process and was particularly indicated to induce and promote pregnancy.

Clary Sage (Salvia sclarea)

Produced in southern France, U.S.S.R., United States.

Distillation of the plant; the oil is clear.

Fragrance: pleasant, sweet with floral notes, slightly musky.

Widely used as a fixative in cosmetics and perfumery.

Organs: Female genitals.

Medicinal Properties and Indications:

Similar to those of Salvia officinalis, with a special emphasis on women's diseases (menstruation, leukorrhea, frigidity.

Clary sage is preferred to the other sages for long cures. (No toxicity).

Sage (*Salvia officinalis*)

Produced in Spain, Yugoslavia, France.
Distillation of leaves and flowers.
Fragrance: harsh, aromatic (*Salvia lavandulifolia*, growing in northern Spain, is finer and milder).
Renowned since antiquity, the "salvia salvatrix" of the Romans is one of the most powerful and versatile medicinal plants. Indeed, *cur moriatur homo, cui salvia crescit in horto?* (why should he die, the one who grows sage in his garden?). That panacea, which preserves health and youth, was always recommended for conception and pregnancy.

Organs: Liver, gallbladder, kidneys.

Medicinal Properties:

Tonic, stimulant (adrenocortical glands, nerves).
Antisudorific.
Antiseptic.
Diuretic.
Emmenagogue.
Hypertensive agent.
Aperitive, stomachic.
Depurative.
Astringent, vulnerary.

Indications:

General weakness, anemmia, asthenia, neurasthenia.
Hypotension.
Sterility, menopause, regulation of menstruation, birth preparation.
Perspiration, fever.
Hepatobiliary and kidney dysfunctions.
Nervous afflictions.
Bronchitis, asthma.
Mouth ulcers, stomatitis, tonsillitis, dermatitis.
Hair loss.
Wounds, ulcers.

The essential oil of sage is tonic at high doses and should not be taken internally for very long. It is not recommended for people with epileptic tendencies.

Thyme (*Thymus vulgaris*)

Produced in Morocco, Spain, France, Greece.
The oil is obtained from branches and flowers. It is a red or brownish-red liquid for the thymol-carvacrol chemotypes and clear to yellowish for the other chemotypes.
Fragrance: Hot, spicy, aromatic for the thymol-carvacrol chemotypes, sweet to fresh and green for the others (citrusy for the citral chemotype, rose-like for the geraniol, etc.).
The genus *Thymus* produces many species, subspecies, and chemotypes all around the Mediterranean sea (see the essential oil quick reference guide at the end of this

book). For some yet unknown reason, the same subspecies produces oils with totally different chemical compositions (this phenomenon, discovered only recently, is called chemotyping). It has been suggested that such variations may be caused by climatic and other environmental conditions. Thus, the burning hot thymol and carvacrol chemotypes would grow at lower altitude and in dryer climates, while the milder geraniol, linalol, citral, and thuyanol chemotypes would grow at higher altitude and milder climates. It has even been suggested that a plant of thyme transplanted from one climatic area to another begins to develop the characteristics of its new location (i.e., a thyme growing in dryness at sea level would be thymol-carvacrol chemotype, but would become linalol or geraniol when transplanted to a higher altitude). As seductive as this theory might be, the reality is slightly different.

There is, in the wild, a predominance of the thymol and carvacrol chemotypes in the dryer and warmer areas, while the milder chemotypes are more abundant under milder conditions. But more than 7 years of wild harvesting of thyme have shown me that the different chemotypes can be found everywhere.

Furthermore, most of the commercial production of chemotyped thymes comes from the same area of southern France, and several farmers grow all the chemotypes on their farms.

Thyme has been widely used for therapy since antiquity for its warming, stimulant, and cleansing properties.

Medicinal Properties:
General stimulant (physic, psychic, capillary circulation).
Antiseptic (lungs, intestine, genitourinary system).
Rubefacient.
Healing.
Balsamic, expectorant.

Indications:
Asthenia, anemia, neurasthenia, nervous deficiency.
Infectious diseases (intestinal and urinary).
Pulmonary diseases (bronchitis, tuberculosis, asthma).
Poor digestion, fermentation.
Rheumatism, arthritis, gout.
Flu, influenza, sore throat.
Wounds.

This tiny bush, with no special requirements for soil quality or the amount of humidity, is quite avid of warmth and light. It is helpful whenever inner warmth is poor or missing: excess of water, chilling tendencies, cold, and weakness of the vital center, especially when it is manifested at the level of lungs or stomach.

Thyme is able to create, by itself, almost the entire spectrum of fragrances demonstrated by the medicinal family: the Labiatae, from the hot burning thymol-carvacrol (reminiscent of oregano or savory) to the citral types similar to melissa, through the linalol types (marjoram, lavender). This shows the amazing adaptability of the genus, its broad-spectrum curative power, and its incredible vital energy. Thymes certainly are among the major oils of aromatherapy.

MYRTACEAE (Harmony; equilibrium in the interaction of the four elements — (fire, air, water, earth)

Essential Oils of the Family: Cajuput, clove, ecualyptus, myrtle, niaouli, nutmeg, tea tree.
Other oils of interest: bay, red pepper.

Myrtaceae grow in the tropical zones of every continent. Confronted with the powerful forces of earth and water in relation to strong tropical influences, Myrtaceae oppose a very structured formating principle.

The plants and trees of the family have a noble and harmonious aspect, which expresses the perfect equilibrium among the four elements in the constitution of the type. The astral sphere is never violent to etheric formating forces: the type does not produce any poisonous plant.

The evergreen leaves are strong and simple. They open themselves to the supra vegetal and animal sphere in an intense floral process (pollination is accomplished by insects and birds). The sugar process is very strong in this family, which produces some delicious fruits: pomegranate, gooseberry, guava, myrtoloela fruits, and jabotica plums.

The deep penetration of tropical warmth into the leaf, the flower, the bark, and the wood generates etheric oils and aromatic resins.

The family also produces some condiments (cloves, red pepper).

Finally, they produce very hard woods, which reveals the healthy relation of this family with the earth element.

Type of Action: Reequilibrating.

Domain of Action: Metabolism, energy centers, lungs.

Indications:
Respiratory diseases.
Metabolic or energetic lack of balance.

Cajuput (*Melaleuca leucadendron*)

Produced in Malaysia and Far Eastern countries.
Distillation of the leaves; the oil is yellowish-green.
Fragrance: penetrating, camphorlike.
Used in numerous pectoral preparations; also used as insecticide and parasiticide.
In Malaysia and Java, cajuput oil was a traditional remedy for cholera and rheumatism.

Medicinal Properties:
General antiseptic (pulmonary, urinary, intestinal).
Antispasmodic, antineuralgic.
Sudorific.
Febrifuge.

Indications:
Pulmonary diseases (bronchitis, tuber-
culosis).
Cystitis, urethritis.
Dysentery, diarrhea, amebiasis.
Rheumatism, rheumatic pains.
Earaches.

Clove (*Eugenia caryophyllata*)

Produced in Molucca Islands, Madagascar,
Zanzibar, Indonesia.
Distillation of the dried buds; the oil is
brown to dark brown.
Clove stems and clove leaves are also distilled; they are of lower quality (especially
the former) and are often used to adulterate clove bud oil.
Fragrance: hot, spicy, characteristic.
Used in dentistry, pharmacy, food industry, perfumery.
Native of the Molucca Islands, clove is one
of the best-known spices in the world, along
with black pepper, cinnamon, and nutmeg.
It was so precious in ancient times that it
caused a few wars: its trade was almost
exclusively controlled by the Portuguese,
who possessed the Molucca Islands until the
seventeenth century, when the Dutch drove
them out. To better control the monopoly
and raise prices, the Dutch destroyed all
plantations except the one on Amboine
Island. The French finally stole a few plants
to start new plantations in Guyana, Zanzibar, Reunion, and Trinidad.
Clove oil was long used in dentistry as an
analgesic.

Medicinal Properties:
Antineuralgic, analgesic.
Powerful antiseptic, cicatrizant.
Stomachic, carminative.
Aphrodisiac, stimulant.
Parasiticide.

Indications:
Toothache.
Prevention of infectious diseases.
Physical and intellectual asthenia (to
strengthen memory).
Dyspepsia, gastric fermentation, flatu-
lence.
Impotence.
Infected wounds, ulcers.

In the clove tree, the terrestrial forces of
the roots rise into the floral area: the essential oil of the buds, heavier than water and
not easily volatile, is heavy and burning,
which reveals that the fire cosmic forces
have been strongly drawn into the ground.
This special interaction of the fire and earth
energies in the floral area results in a strong
action on the metabolism: clove stimulates
the digestion of heavy food and regulates the
digestive tract.

Eucalyptus (*Eucalyptus globulus*)

Produced in Australia, Spain, Portugal.
Distillation of the leaves; the oil is yellow
to red.
Fragrance; fresh, balsamic, camphorlike.
Numerous uses in pharmacy.

Native of Australia, where it was regarded as a general cure-all by the Aborigines and later by the white settlers, eucalyptus has now spread almost entirely over the tropical and subtropical parts of the world. It has a long tradition of uses in medicine, and its essential oil is one of the most powerful and versatile remedies.

Medicinal Properties:
General antiseptic (especially pulmonary and urinary).
Balsamic, expectorant, antispasmodic.
Hypoglycemic.
Febrifuge.
Stimulant.
Cicatrizant, vulnerary.
Parasiticide.

Indications:
Respiratory diseases (asthma, bronchitis, tuberculosis, flu, sinusitis).
Urinary infections.
Diabetes.
Fevers.
Rheumatism.
Intestinal parasites (ascaris, oxyurids).

One of the tallest trees in the world, eucalyptus is also deeply rooted: its roots go amazingly deep in the ground to find aquifer veins and strongly draw water to its vigorous branches and leaves. It is used to drain marshy areas and cleanse them from mosquitoes. It grows incredibly fast, but forms nevertheless a very strong wood, fairly resistant to rot. The leaves, shaped like swords, are oriented in such a way as to avoid a strong exposure to the sun, and allow the light to go through the whole tree and reach the ground. Eucalyptus energetically draws the solidifying forces of earth and water into the clear and dry area of air and light, where it attracts astral forces for the production of essential oils—hence its action on the urinary and pulmonary systems. It is especially beneficent in the treatment of pulmonary inflammation and excessive mucosity.

Myrtle (*Myrtus communis*)

Produced in North Africa
Distillation of branches; the oil is yellow.
Fragrance: fresh, close to eucalyptus.

The Greeks and Romans used myrtle for pulmonary and urinary diseases. In the sixteenth century, the leaves and flowers were used for skin care; they served in the preparation of "angel water," a renowned tonic and astringent lotion.

Specific Therapetuic Indications:
Skin care.
The medicinal properties of myrtle closely resemble those of eucalyptus.

Niaouli (*Melaleuca viridiflora*)

Produced in Madagascar, Australia, and New Caledonia.
Distillation of the leaves; the oil (also called "gomenol") is yellow.

Fragrance: strong, camphorlike, balsamic, close to eucalyptus.

Same medicinal properties and indications as eucalyptus.

Specific Therapeutic Indications:
Stimulating to tissues (promotes local circulation and leukocyte and antibody activity).

Infected wounds, ulcers, burns.

Nutmeg (*Myristica fragrans*; Myristicaceae)

Produced in the West Indies, Indonesia, Java.

Distillation of the nuts; the oil is colorless.

The nut is surrounded by a fleshy shell, which, by distillation, yields an essential oil called mace oil; it is of lower quality than nutmeg oil, with similar composition and properties.

Fragrance: spicy, peppery, aromatic.

Some applications in pharmaceutical preparations; few uses in perfumery; widely used for the manufacture of spirits and elixirs.

First mentioned in the fifth century, nutmeg was introduced to the Occident by Arabian merchants. Portugal had the monopoly of its trade until 1605, when the Dutch took over their possessions. The plantations were placed under military protection, and prices were kept high by systematic destruction of the trees growing in nearby islands. Huge amounts of the spice were even burned at intervals to keep the price high. Pierre Poivre finally stole a few plants in 1768, and the nutmeg tree was then grown in other tropical countries.

Nutmeg has been highly appreciated since the early middle ages and was an ingredient of numerous balms, elixirs, and unguents. In 1704, Pollini wrote more than 800 pages on the invaluable virtues of nutmeg! He concluded, "in good health or disabled, alive or dead, nobody can do without this nut, the most salutary medicine!"

It is indeed a very powerful tonic and stimulant.

Organs: Digestive system.

Medicinal Properties:
Tonic, stimulant (nervous system, circulation).

Digestive, intestinal antiseptic.

Sedative, analgesic.

Aphrodisiac.

Stupefying and toxic at high doses (delirim, hallucinations, fainting).

Indications:
Digestive problems, intestinal infections, flatulence.

Asthenia.

Nervous and intellectual fatigue.

Impotence.

Rheumatic pain, neuralgia.

Tea Tree (*Melaleuca alternifolia*)

Produced in Australia.

Distillation of leaves; the oil is yellowish.

Fragrance: strong, camphorlike, balsamic, pungent.

A relative newcomer on the aromatherapy scene, tea tree has quickly become a universal panacea, first-aid kit, or cure-all. It is (with oregano and savory) one of the oils whose medical and antiseptic properties are the most widely documented. Researches started in the late 1920s in Australia and showed the amazing antiinfectious power of the oil. During World War II, it was even included in military first-aid kits in tropical areas. Extensive research during the 1970s and 1980s has showed its strong antifungus action (Morton Walker, Dr. Eduardo F. Pena, Dr. Paul Belaiche). Its wide range of action and its low toxicity make it an ideal home remedy for inclusion in any aromatherapy first-aid kit (with lavender and eucalyptus).

Medicinal Properties:
Antifungus (*Candida albicans, Trichomonas*).
Antiinfectious.
General antiseptic (especially urinary).
Immunostimulant.
Balsamic, expectorant.
Cicatrizant, vulnerary.
Parasiticide.

Indications:
Fungal infections (ringworm, athlete's foot, vaginitis, thrush, *Candida albicans*).
Urinary infections, cystitis.
Infected wounds, ulcers, sores, and any infectious condition.
Cold sores, blisters, chickenpox.
Acne.
Rashes, anal and genital pruritis, genital herpes.
Intestinal parasites.
Surgery preparation (prevention).
Low immune system.
Dandruff, hair care.

A somewhat small tree with needle-type leaves (similar to cypress), tea tree shows an amazing vitality. Before becoming a rare commodity when the demand for its oil increased dramatically in the 1980s, tea tree was considered a weed—a real plague, in fact—and farmers could not get rid of it. Cut down to the roots, it grows flourishing, thick foliage in less than 2 years. Even more than eucalyptus, it likes swampy, marshy areas. Unlike eucalyptus, though, its leaves are hardly developed, which indicates a predominance of earth, fire, and water over air. Tea tree yields one of the best antifungus, antiinfectious, and antiseptic oils, but eucalyptus works better on respiratory conditions. Finally, the amazing vitality of tea tree indicates its strong immunostimulant properties.

PEPPER (*Piper nigrum*; Piperaceae)

Produced in India, Java, Sumatra, China.
Distillation of the seeds; the oil is yellow-green.
Fragrance: characteristic.
Few uses in perfumery and food industry.

One of the most ancient spices, pepper was mentioned in Chinese and Sanskrit texts a few thousand years ago. In the Western countries, it was the most valued spice, and was used as currency in the Middle Ages. The essential oil of pepper is described by Valerius Cordius in his *Compendium Aromatorium* in 1488. It is traditionally indicated as a stimulant, tonic, and whenever there is an excess of cold or water.

Medicinal Properties:
Stimulant, tonic (especially digestive and nervous systems).
Digestive, stomachic, antitoxic.
Heating, drying, comforting.
Analgesic, rubefacient.
Aphrodisiac.
Stimulant of the root chakra.

Indications:
Digestive problems (dyspepsia, flatulence, loss of appetite, food poisoning).
Fever, cold, catarrh, cough, influenza.
Neuralgia, toothache, rheumatic aches.
Muscular pain, sport massage (preparation for effort).
Gonorrhea.
Impotence.
Ungroundedness.

ROSE (*Rosa centifolia* and *damascena;* Rosaceae)

Produced in Bulgaria, Morocco, Turkey.
The rose buds are picked for a few hours only, in the morning, right after the dew, and distilled immediately; the oil is rather thick, yellow to greenish-yellow.
Fragrance: characteristic.
One of the most expensive essential oils, rose oil is almost always adulterated with substances like geranium, lemongrass, palmarosa, and terpene alcohols (geraniol, citronellol, rhodinol, linalol, nerol, etc.). The processes of adulteration have become so refined that it is almost impossible to disclose the frauds.
Real rose oil is only used in very high-grade perfumes.
Rose water is widely used in cosmetics and perfumery.
Whether it sprang from the blood of Venus, the blood of Adonis, or the sweat of Mohammed, the rose—the queen of flowers—is certainly immemorial. Praised by the poets, revered in the sacred books, and offered to the kings and the gods, the rose is a traditional symbol of love.
Bunches of roses were found in the sarcophagus of Tutankhamon, offered by the Queen Ankhsenamon as a token of her love. When the Persian Emperor Djihanguyr married the Princess Nour-Djihan, a canal encircling the gardens was filled with rose water. Droplets of oil were noticed floating on top of the water; that was the beginning of the production of the famous Persian rose oil.

Organs & Functions: Female reproductive system, heart chakra.

Medicinal Properties:
Uplifting, antidepressant, tonic.

Astringent, hemostatic.
Depurative.
Aphrodisiac.
Stimulant of the heart chakra.

Indications:

Nervous tension, depression, insomnia, headache.

Skin care (wrinkles, eczema, sensitive skin, aged skin).

Disorders of the female reproductive system: frigidity, sterility, uterine dissorders.

Hemorrhage.

Impotence.

Emotional shock, grief, depression.

Rose water is an excellent skin tonic, recommended for any type of skin; it is good for wrinkles, inflammation, redness, sensitive skins. Indicated for ophthalmia.

ROSEWOOD (*Aniba roseaodora*; Lauraceae)

Produced in Brazil.

Distillation of the chopped wood; the oil is clear to pale yellow.

Fregrance: very sweet, floral, woody. Blends very well with almost any oil.

Rosewood oil is one of the major oils of perfumery, where it is used as a middle note. It was little used in aromatherapy until recently. Although it does not have any dramatic curative power (like tea tree or lavender), I find it very useful, especially for skin care. It is very mild and safe to use. It is also a very useful oil in blending, and helps to give body to a blend and to round sharp edges.

Medicinal Properties:

Cellular stimulant, tissue regenerator.
Uplifting, antidepressant, tonic.
Calming, cephalic.

Indications:

Headache nausea.

Skin care (sensitive skin, aged skin, wrinkles, general skin care).

Scars, wounds.

Rosewood is excellent for any type of body care or skin care preparation (bath oils, lotions, masks, facials).

RUTACEAE (Processes of subdued tropical heat)

Essential Oils of the Family: Bergamot, grapefruit, lemon, lime, neroli, orange, petitgrain, tangerine.

Other oils of interest: rue (*Ruta graveolens*). Warning: this oil is highly toxic and should be used with great care.

Most Rutaceae grow in the tropical area; in these areas, they are mostly small thorny trees with hard wood which is often resinous, and firm green leaves. Their beautiful abundant flowers shaped like symmetrical stars exhale a delicious, sweet, slightly exhilarating fragrance. The scent of the leaves is fresh and comforting with a hint of bitterness. The trees develop juicy acid fruits (citrus) or small, hot, spicy berries.

The general therapeutic activity of the type concerns the interaction of warmth and fluid in the body. The oils reduce pro- liferations, distensions, inflammations, and looseness; they strengthen the astral body, and their formating forces are activated by air and warmth.

Type of Action:
Cooling, refreshing.
Sedative (flowers).
Control of liquid processes, secretion (fruits).

Domain of Action:
Digestive system, kidneys, liver.
Nervous system.

Indications:
Inflammations, infectious diseases.
Excess of liquids (obesity).
Oversensitivity, nervous tension.

The Genus *Citrus*

Neroli essential oil is obtained by distillation of the flowers.

Distillation of the leaves gives petitgrain.

The essential oils of bergamot; grapefruit, lemon, lime, orange, and tangerine are extracted from the peel of the fruits by cold pressure.

Extremely prolific (each tree can produce up to 100 fruits), deeply rooted, and densely ramified, citruses perfectly control the interaction of the two powerful opposite flows of forces: centrifugal forces that strongly draw up the terrestrial forces, charging them with vitalized fluid elements of a tropical luxuriance, and cosmic forces of light and warmth that are absorbed by the leaves, the bark, the wood, and the fruit. Their energetic floral process and their light, suave, almost ethereal and very pervasive fragrance suggest an etheric organism intensely penetrated by the peripheral astral sphere. Citrus fruits are liquid like a berry, but are surrounded with a tough envelope shaped by the forces of air and warmth.

Citruses then strive against the dissolving centrifugal forces of the tropical world. Their action is refreshing, vivifying, and tonic, and tends to gather the constitutive elements of the body.

The floral area expresses a soft, delicious, appeasing exhilaration, indicative of the remarkable sedative, antidepressant power of the blossoms. The fragrance of the thick, vigorous leaves is less refined, more hearty and grounded, and slightly bitter. Their action is then invigorating, comforting, and almost materialistic, even compared with the ethereal neroli.

Bergamot (*Citrus bergamia*)

Produced in Italy, Ivory Coast, Guinea.

Cold pressure of the rind of the fruit; the oil is yellowish-green, emerald.

Fragrance; sweet, citrusy, with floral note.

Widely used in perfumery; blends perfectly with almost any oil; makes a perfect top note.

Medicinal Properties:
Antispasmodic.

Antiseptic.

Cordial, tonic, stomachic, digestive.

Vulnerary.

Indications:
Colic, intestinal infection, intestinal parasites, stomatitis.

Skin care.

Grapefruit (*Citrus paradisi*)

Mostly produced in the United States.

Various uses in perfumery and food industry.

Blends fairly well with other citrus oils, geranium, cedarwood.

Specific Therapeutic Indications:
Obesity.

Lemon (*Citrus limonum*)

Produced all around the Mediterranean and in California, Brazil, and Argentina.

Extraction by cold pressure of the skin; the oil is yellow to yellowish-green.

Numerous uses in perfumery, cosmetics, pharmacy, and the food and soap industries.

Blends well with many oils; makes a nice green note.

One of the most versatile essential oils in aromatherapy.

Medicinal Properties:
Bactericide, antiseptic, stimulant of leukocytosis.

Stimulant, tonic.

Stomachic, carminative.

Diuretic.

Hepatic.

Liquefy the blood, hypothensive agent.

Depurative.

Antirheumatic.

Indications:
Infectious diseases.

Anemia, asthenia.

Varicosis, arteriosclerosis, hyperviscosity of the blood, hypertension.

Rheumatism.

Dyspepsia, flatulence.

Hepatic congestion.

Skin diseases, skin care.

Herpes.

Profusely thorny, with very thick leaves and the most acid fruit of the vegetable kingdom, the small lemon tree gives an impression of fresh, optimistic, fearless strength. Here the fire/water dialectic is resolved on the cooling side. The fruit is tightly structured under a fairly tough skin; expansion, dilation, and inflation are under control.

Lime (*Citrus limetta*)

Produced in Florida, Central America, Caribbean Islands.

The oil is extracted from the skin by cold pressure or distillation. The cold-pressed oil is far superior to the distilled oil; it is gold to yellowish-green.

Fragrance: fresh, green, very pleasant; similar to bergamot for the cold-pressed oil; much heavier for the distilled oil.

The indications and various uses of lime are similar to those of lemon (although its refreshing quality is more pronounced). Makes a very good after-shave lotion.

Neroli (Orange Blossom; *Citrus vulgaris*)

Real neroli (also called neroli biguarade) is extracted from bitter orange blossom (or *biguarade*). However, other citrus blossoms are sometimes distilled (sweet orange, lemon, mandarin).

Produced in France, Spain, North Africa, Italy, and recently, the Comoro Islands.

One of the most expensive oils, therefore widely adulterated.

Fragrance: one of the finest floral essences; sweet, suave, delicious, slightly euphoric.

Used in expensive cologne and perfumes, it blends well with almost any oil and is useful as the heart of a floral blend.

Native of China, where its flowers were traditionally used in cosmetics, orange trees now grow all around the Mediterranean, in the United States, and in Central and South America.

Neroli was already being produced in the beginning of the sixteenth century. It became a fashionable perfume when the Duchess of Nerole started using it to scent her gloves.

Medicinal Properties:

Antidepressant, antispasmodic, sedative.
Diminishes the amplitude of heart muscle contractions.
Aphrodisiac.
Stimulant of the heart chakra.

Indications:

Insomnia, hysteria, anxiety, depression, nervous tension.
Palpitations.
Diarrhea related to stress.
Skin care (dry or sensitive skin).
Grief, emotional shock.
The hydrolate obtained by distillation is more commonly known as orange-flower water; it is widely used for skin care and pastry-making.
It is soothing, digestive, carminative.
Mild remedy for infants' colics and to send them to sleep.

Orange (*Citrus auranthium*)

Produced in Spain, North Africa, United States, and Central and South America.

The oil is orange.

Numerous uses in perfumery and food industry.

Medicinal Properties:

Febrifuge.
Stomachic, digestive.
Antispasmodic, sedative, cardiotonic.

Indications:

Fever.
Indigestion, dyspepsia, flatulence, gastric spasms.

Skin care, wrinkles, dermatitis. Nervous troubles.

Biguarade, or bitter orange, is even more thorny than lemon; the strong bitterness of its fruit indicates a special affinity for the liver.

With sweet orange, qualities are softened: no more thorns, and the fruit is now totally edible. The water processes are no longer so tight. The soothing properties are more pronounced.

Petitgrain (Bitter Orange Leaves)

Like neroli, real petitgrain (or petitgrain biguarade) is obtained by distilling the leaves of the bitter orange tree. Petitgrain bergamot, petitgrain lemon, and petitgrain mandarin are also produced.

Areas of production: same as neroli.

Fragrance: fresh, invigorating, slightly floral with a bitter note.

Widely used in pharmacy and perfumery (the basic ingredient of good colognes). Blends well with almost any oil.

Specific Therapeutic Indications:
Painful digestion, sedative of nervous system.
Tonic, intellectual stimulant, strengthen memory.

Tangerine (Citrus reticulata)

Produced in Italy (mandarin) and United States (tangerine).

Mandarin oil is much finer than tangerine oil (a hybrid).

Fragrance: sweeter than orange, reminiscent of bergamot.

Native of China, tangerine is the most delicate citrus fruit; it was traditionally offered to the mandarins (hence the name mandarin). The medicinal properties of tangerine are very close to those of orange. The sedative and antispasmodic properties, however, are more pronounced.

Specific Therapeutic Indications: Calming, antispasmodic, slightly, hypnotic nervous tension, insomnia, epilepsy).

Mandarin is certainly the softest of all citrus trees. The leaves are delicate, the fruit is very sweet, and the taste is quite refined. The peel is soft and the fragrance is almost exotic. The soothing action on the nervous centers is then quite pronounced.

SANDALWOOD (Santalum albumu; Santalaceae)

Produced in India, Indonesia, and China.

Distillation of the inner wood; the oil is thick and yellow.

Fragrance: characteristic (persistent, woody, sweet, spicy, oriental).

Very good fixative, widely used in high-class perfumes. Often adulterated.

A sacred tree of India, sandalwood is mentioned in the old Sanskrit and Chinese books. It was widely used as incense, in religious ceremonies, and in medicine and cosmetics.

Organs: Genitourinary tract.

Medicinal Properties:
Genitourinary antiseptic, diuretic.
Antidepressant, tonic, aphrodisiac.
Antispasmodic.
Astringent.

Indications:
Genitourinary infections: gonorrhea, blenorrhea, cystitis, colibacillosis.
Impotence.

UMBELLIFERAE (Plants of the Air Element)

Essential Oils of the Family: Angelica, aniseed, caraway, carrot, coriander, cumin, fennel, lovage.

Other oils of interest: ammi-visnaga, aneth, asafetida, celery, galbanum, parsley.

This family is characterized by the extreme division of the leaves, ending up in an aerial explosion in such plants as fennel or anise. The leaf is the organ of interaction and confrontation between air and water, light and darkness. Umbelliferae obviously are very sensitive to this confrontation. The interaction of air, light, water, and earth through these extremely ramified leaves gives birth, in a contraction process, to a strong root or vigorous rhizome, which stays underground for one year or more. This subterranean organ draws the cosmic forces into the ground. Then vegetation grows rapidly in a radiating explosion, until it reaches the final bouquet of the inflorescence, with its radiating umbel – each branch of the umbel splitting again in umbellules.

The special interaction of this family with the air element is further emphasized by their ability to incorporate air within themselves in hollow stems, hollow seeds, and even hollow rhizomes.

In the archetypal plant, the interaction between the plant's etheric organism and the surrounding astral forces takes place in the flower area. This process is manifested in the colors and fragrance of the flower and the formation of nectar. Umbelliferae attract cosmic forces in the leaves, the stem, and even the rhizome. Their aromatic substances are therefore heavier, harsher, and less refined than floral scents.

Umbelliferae, in fact, start their fructification process in the leaves, or even the root. They produce some of the most tasty vegetables (carrot, celery, fennel) and condiments (parsley, coriander, chervil, anise, cumin, carvi, etc.).

In addition to this descending movement, there is also an ascending movement of mucilages and gums, another characteristic of the family.

The therapeutic action of Umbelliferae is then easy to understand. First of all, they have an obvious affinity for the digestive system (especially the intestine). There is also a strong action on the secretions and the glandular system. Finally, they are useful in respiratory diseases. According to Robert Tisserand in *Aromatherapy to Heal and Tend the Body*, "tissue regeneration in the livers of rats has been demonstrated with essential oils, in particular the four seed oils—cumin, fennel, celery and parsley" (which all belong to the Umbelliferae family). Carrot seed oil has been used successfully to fight the aging skin process.

Type of Action:
Accumulation/excretion, elimination.
Secretion (diuretic, sudorific, expectorant).
Regulation of the aerial processes in the organism (carminative, antispasmodic).
Tissue regeneration.

Domain of Action:
Digestive system (especially intestines), glandular system.
Respiratory system.

Indications:
Digestive and intestinal problems, accumulation of gas.
Spasms (digestive, respiratory, circulatory).
Glandular problems.

Angelica (*Angelica archangelica*)

Produced in Belgium, France, Poland.
The oil is obtained from seeds or roots; it is almost colorless.
Fragrance: balsamic, nicely aromatic, slightly musky.

Several varieties of angelica grow in northern Europe; the main ones are *Angelica sylvestris* (wild) and *Angelica archangelica* (domestic, cultured). The plant was highly valued by the physician of the Renaissance. Paracelsus reported that it was of great help during the epidemic of pestilence in Milan in 1510.

Medicinal Properties:
Depurative, sudorific.
Stomachic, digestive, aperitive.
Stimulant, tonic, cephalic, revitalizing.

Indications:
Nervous afflictions related to the digestive system (cramps, spasms, aerophagia, digestive migraine).
Weakness of stomach.
Asthenia, anemia, anorexia, rachitis, neurovegetative cardiopathies.
Lung diseases (bronchitis, flu, pneumonia, pleuresy).
Gout (compresses, massage).

This vigorous prolific plant of the air element (with a hollow stem) grows in deep humid soils and rather cool temperate climates. (It grows wild by streams and irrigation canals.) Therefore, it is a typical plant of elimination. It helps to eliminate toxins, purify the blood and lymph, and stimulate the glandular system. It is recommended for weakness and nervousness, and for convalescents and old people.

Aniseed (*Pimpinella anisum*)

Produced in Spain, Egypt, North Africa, U.S.S.R.
Distillation of the seeds; the oil is slightly yellow.

Mentioned in the Vedas and the Bible, anise was considered one of the main medicinal plants in China, India, Egypt, Greece, and Rome. According to Pythagorus, it is an excellent carminative and appetizer.

Medicinal Properties:
Stomachic, carminative, antispasmodic.
General stimulant (digestive, respiratory, cardiac).
Galactagogue.
Diuretic.
Aphrodisiac.
Stupefying at high doses.

Indications:
Nervous dyspepsia, aerophagia, gas accumulation, digestive migraines.
Insufficient milk (nursing mothers).
Impotence, frigidity.
Epilepsy.

Unlike most Umbelliferae, anise grows flowers and seeds in its first year. Only in a very dry climate can the seeds fully ripen. The forces of warmth are thus condensed in these small aniseeds, the taste of which is aqueous and fiery. The medicinal properties of anise are then the same as of most plants of the type, but its antispasmodic expectorant power is accentuated, with a narcotic or even stupefying effect.

Caraway (*Carum carvi*)

Produced in northern Europe.
Distillation of seeds; oil is yellowish.

Caraway seed is used in pastries and delicatessen foods in northern Europe and the Arab countries. Its medicinal properties are very close to these of aniseed.

Medicinal Properties:
Carminative.
Antispasmodic.
General stimulant (digestive, respiratory, cardiac).
Diuretic.

Indications:
Digestive and intestinal troubles.
Aerophagia, gas accumulation, fermentations.
Nervous dyspepsia, digestive migraine.
Scabies, mange (dogs) (see Valnet).

Carrot (*Daucus carota*)

Produced in France, Egypt, India.
Distillation of the seeds; the oil is slightly yellow.
Fragrance: characteristic (carrot-like).

Carrot has been used since the sixteenth century as a carminative, diuretic, and hepatic, and for skin diseases.

Medicinal Properties:
Depurative, hepatic.
Emmenagogue.
Diuretic.

Indications:
Jaundice, hepatobiliary disorders.

Favors menstruation and conception. Skin diseases.

Coriander (*Coriandrum sativum*)

Produced in North Africa, Spain, U.S.S.R.
Distillation of the seeds; the oil is slightly yellow.
Fragrance: anisey, musky, aromatic.

Seeds of coriander found in Egyptian sepulchers prove that it was already used by the time of Ramses II. Theophrasta, Hippocrates, Galen and Pliny talk about its properties as stimulant, carminative, and digestive.

Medicinal Properties and Indications:
Same as all Umbelliferae (aerophagia, digestion, flatulence, spasms).
Stupefying at high doses.

Cumin (*Cuminum cyminum*)

Produced in North Africa and the Far East.
Distillation of the seeds; the oil is slightly yellow.
Fragrance: bitter, anisey, aromatic.

Native of Egypt, cumin is a close relative of coriander. It was a traditional spice in the Middle East and is one of the ingredients of curry. It is an excellent digestive stimulant, which should however be used with great care, as it can provoke skin irritation.

Medicinal Properties and Indications:
Same as all Umbelliferae (aerophagia, digestion, flatulence, spasms).

Fennel (*Foeniculum vulgare*)

Produced in Spain, North Africa, India, Japan.
Distillation of the seeds; the oil is yellowish.
Fragrance: strong, anisey, camphoric.

Used in India, Egypt, China. In the Middle Ages, people used it to prevent witchcraft and as a protection against evil spirits.

Medicinal Properties:
Aperitive, stomachic, carminative.
Emmenagogue, galactagogue.
Diuretic.
Antispasmodic.
Laxative.

Indications:
Dyspepsia, flatulence, digestive problems, aerophagia.
Amenorrhea, menopausal problems.
Insufficient milk.
Oliguria, obesity, kidney stones.

Lovage (*Levisticum officinalis*)

Produced in France and Belgium.
Distillation of the roots; the oil is slightly yellow.
Fragrance: musky, earthy.

Medicinal Properties:
  Intestinal and kidney stimulant.
  Diuretic.
  Drainer, detoxifier.

Indications:
  Kidney afflictions (cystitis, nephritis, albuminuria, etc.).
  Water retention; edema.
  Intestinal fermentation.

VERBENA (Lemon Verbena) (*Lippia citriodora*; Verbenaceae)

Produced in southern France and North Africa.

Distillation of the branches; the oil is yellowish-green.

Fragrance: fresh and lemony, similar to lemongrass but more refined.

There is much confusion about this oil; many essential oils are improperly called verbena. Indian verbena is a variety of lemongrass, while exotic verbena is Litsea cubeba, both plants from the Graminae family (cf. these plants in the Graminae section).

Native of Chile and Peru, true lemon verbena is a small bush with an abundant leaf system. The leaves are steam distilled for the production of the oil. The yield is very low, making true lemon verbena oil rather rare and expensive. The world production of the oil is limited and represents only a tiny fraction of the sale of the oil (I'll let you guess where the rest comes from).

True lemon verbena is a lovely oil that gives a nice fresh, lemony top note to blends. It is best used in the diffuser.

Medicinal Properties:
  Liver and digestive stimulant.
  Cooling, refreshing, febrifuge.
  Neurovegetative system.
  Calming at low doses.

Indications:
  Nervousness, insomnia, tachycardia.
  Digestive troubles.

YLANG YLANG (*Unona odorantissimum*; Anonaceae)

Ylang ylang is closley related to cananga (*Canaga odorata*). The two could in fact be the same tree; the slight difference between the essences would then depend on the country of production and the method of distillation.

Produced in Reunion, the Comoro Islands, Madagascar, Java, Sumatra, Philippines.

The distillation of the flowers is a delicate operation, which lasts for days; it yields up to six different qualities, from extra-superior to fifth grade. The "complete" (i.e., the whole oil) should be used for aromatherapy. The oil is yellowish and syrupy.

Fragrance: sweet, voluptuous, exotic (even sickening for some people).

It makes a good fixative.

Ylang ylang, which means "flower of flowers," is a tree growing up to 60 feet high that produces beautiful yellow flowers. In

Indonesia, people spread them on the bed of newly married couples on their wedding night. In the Molucca Islands, people soak ylang ylang and cucuma flowers in coconut oil to prepare a ointment called borri-borri that they use for skin care, hair care, and skin diseases, and to prevent fever.

According to R. W. Moncrieff, "ylang ylang oil soothes and inhibits anger born of frustration."

Medicinal Properties:
Hypotensive.
Aphrodisiac.
Antidepressant, sedative, euphoric.
Antiseptic (for intestinal infections).

Indications:
Tachycardia, palpitations.
Hypertension, hyperpnea.
Depression, nervous tension, insomnia.
Impotence, frigidity.
Skin care.

Supremely exotic, ylang ylang has the soothing, sedative, slightly euphoric, even lascivious quality of extreme fire and water, the luxurious laziness of tropical islands. It is used especially as a perfume, in baths, for massage, and in cosmetics. It also has a soothing effect on the skin and is recommended for oily skin.

EIGHT

The Art of Blending

As I have mentioned before, aromatherapy acts on different levels. On the physical level, essential oils can cure most of the common diseases. Essential oils also have a profound action on the energy level and they deeply affect the emotions and the psyche. More importantly, aromatherapy has a definitive playful, Dionisiac dimension to it; it is joyful, lightening, and heartening. Unlike heavy-duty therapy in which you have to suffer first in order to deserve your recovery, enjoyment is part of the aromatic treatment!

Blending is a very important part of aromatherapy. It allows one to give precise and accurate treatments, and also adds to the fun and lightness. Blending is the creative part of aromatherapy; it is an art. Like any art, it requires a balance of practice and intuition. There are some basic rules, but the rules will not create masterpiece without the proper dose of intuition.

Nature offers hundreds of essential oils.

More practically, you can readily find on the marketplace 50–80 of the most common oils (such as lavender, eucalyptus, lemon, bergamot, cedarwood, and ylang ylang) and some more exotic and unusual ones (such as cistus, everlasting, lovage, and melissa). There are now in this country some very reputable sources offering a wide selection of oils (see resource guide). But through blending, you have access to infinite variations.

THE CONCEPT OF SYNERGY

Like almost anything that is influenced by life forces, aromatherapy does not abide by mathematical law. The whole is not the sum of its parts: 2 plus 2 does not equal 4; it might equal 3 or 5, or sometimes even 10! Whenever the whole is greater than the sum of its parts, it is called a synergy. Some essential oils have mutually enhancing power, while others may have inhibiting power on each other. The combination of mutually enhancing oils is a synergy. Synergies allow the therapist to be accurate in treatment.

Creating synergies is a most important part of blending. It requires a deep understanding of the essential oils, a fair amount of experience, and a lot of intuition. Besides, synergies are context-dependent. A given combination of oils may be an excellent synergy for one patient but not appropriate for another.

In order to create a good synergy, you must take into account not only the symptom to be treated but also the underlying cause of the disorder, the biological terrain, and the psychological or emotional factors involved.

All this may sound discouraging to the beginner, but if you follow a few basic rules, you will be able to create good blends.

First of all, do not blend more than three or four oils at a time until you have gained enough experience.

Do not blend oils with opposite effects (like a calming oil and a stimulant oil).

Check thoroughly the properties of the oils that you want to blend, and make sure that they complement each other for the particular patient that you want to treat.

Finally, a blend has to be pleasant to your patient. This may well be the most important part of blending. Once you have selected the oils that will be efficient for your patient, look at their fragrance compatibility and adjust your blend accordingly.

I will give below some basic rules of thumb for proportion, as well as some basic blends that can be used advantageously for common ailments.

THE PRINCIPLES OF BLENDING

For blending purposes, essential oils are classified into top notes, middle notes, and base notes. A good perfume composition should harmoniously balance these three categories of fragrances.

I have added my own classification into modifiers, enhancers, and equalizers. In work with fragrances, any classification is bound to be highly subjective. Different authors may disagree about the classification of certain oils. Although in many parts of this book I systematically checked my information against other people's findings, here I mostly relied on my own knowledge and experience of the oils to establish the classifications. I encourage my readers to do the same as soon as their own experience will allow. Such classifications are mere tools and should be used as such. If you find a better one, do not hesitate to use it.

Top Notes

Top notes will hit you first in a fragrance. They do not last very long, but they are very important in a blend, as they give the first impression of the blend. Typical top notes are bergamot, petitgrain, neroli, lemon, lime, orange (all citruses in fact), lemongrass, peppermint, thyme, cinnamon, and clove.

Top notes are sharp, penetrating, volatile, extreme, and either cold or hot, but never warm.

While certain top notes can be used rather liberally (lemon, bergamot, petitgrain), the sharpest ones should be used in very small amounts (cinnamon, clove, thyme).

Middle Notes

Middle notes give body to blends; they smooth the sharp edges and round the angles. Typical middle notes are rosewood, geranium, lavender, chamomile, and marjoram. They are warm, round, soft, and mellow. They often are blend enhancers (see below); that is, oils that are added to the blend not so much for their medicinal properties as for their fragrant qualities.

Middle notes typcially form the bulk of the blend (50% and up to 80%).

Base Notes

Base notes (or fixatives) deepen your blend and draw it into the skin, giving it roots and permanence. Typical base notes are cistus, clary sage, patchouli, myrrh, frankincense, cedarwood, and vetiver. When smelled from the bottle, base notes may seem rather faint, but when applied to the skin, they strongly react and release their power, which lasts for several hours, or even days for the animal fixatives such as musk or civet.

The first hit of a fixative is not necessarily very pleasant (musk and civet are defin-

itely obnoxious, while patchouli is unpleasant to many people and vetiver or cistus seems rather weird), but no decent perfume could be made without them. They should be used rather sparingly, so as not to overpower the blend (they rarely account for more than 5% of any blend). Finally, while they are not really necessary to a diffuser blend (though they add depth to it), they are almost mandatory in any preparation to be applied to the skin.

Base notes are deep, intense, profound. Most of them have traditional ritual uses. They generally affect the chakras and have deep effects on the mental, emotional, and spiritual plane and on the astral body.

Essential oils have rather complex chemical composition, and therefore many oils have notes in several categories. Certain oils even cover the whole spectrum from top note to base note. This is the case for ylang ylang or jasmine (with a predominance in the middle and base notes), and for rose (with a predominance in the top and middle notes). Since such oils are most balanced, it is not surprising that they are the most pleasant that nature has to offer. They can in fact be used by themselves as perfumes.

Blend Equalizers

Blend equalizers are those oils that allow you to get rid of the sharp edges. They fill the gaps and help your blend flow harmoniously. They control the intensity of your most active ingredients.

Most of the blend equalizers are context-dependent—that is, they will perform better with certain types of blends.

Rosewood and wild Spanish marjoram are universal equalizers.

Orange and tangerine are excellent with other citruses (neroli, petitgrain, bergamot), spices (clove, cinnamon, nutmeg), and floral fragrances (ylang ylang, jasmine, rose, geranium).

Fir and pine greatly improve blends of Myrtaceae or Coniferae.

The main purpose of the blend equalizers is to hold the blend together but to have little effect on its distinctive personality. They can be used in fairly large amounts (up to 50%), especially in those blends where you need to use some of the sharpest oils.

They are also used advantageously with the most precious oils (such as rose, jasmine, neroli, and melissa).

Blend Modifiers (or Personifiers)

The most intense fragrances (such as clove, cinnamon, peppermint, thyme, blue chamomile, cistus, patchouli) should be used rather sparingly (not more than 2% or 3%).

Such essential oils have the power to greatly affect the overall fragrant quality of your blends, even when used in very small amounts (as low as a fraction of 1%). They are found at each end of the spectrum and are responsible for the sharp edges or the deep roots. They are also the ones that give your blend that very special kick and contribute to its distinctive personality (but one extra drop or two might kill it).

If your blend is rather flat and uninteresting, adding such an oil—at your own risk, and drop by drop, please—may improve it.

Blend Enhancers

Between the modifiers and the equalizers are found the enhancers. Bergamot, cedarwood, geranium, clary sage, lavender, lemon, lime, *Litsea cubeba*, palmarosa, sandalwood, spruce, ylang ylang, and (for the precious oils) jasmine, rose, neroli, and myrrh belong to this category.

Oils like cajeput, eucalyptus, niaouli, and rosemary could be placed into this category, although they are used best in blends for inhalation (diffuser, sauna, steam room).

Such oils have a pleasant fragrance by themselves. They have enough personality to modify your blend and give it a personal touch, while they will not overpower it if used in a reasonable amount. Enhancers may amount to up to 50% of your blend, each individual oil rarely accounting for more than 15% of it.

DOSES AND PROPORTIONS FOR SOME BASIC PREPARATIONS

Once you have prepared your blend, you will use it straight only for inhalation purposes (diffuser, sauna, steam room).

For most other purposes, you will need to add some of your blend to a carrier. The following suggestions will help you determine the proper dosage for the most common preparations.

Massage oil: For full body massage.
   50 drops blend in 4 oz. carrier oil.

Massage oil concentrate: To massage a local area, such as lower back, hips, legs; such a dosage is indicated for treatment of conditions such as cellulitis, rheumatism, sports injuries abdominal cramps, etc.
   50 drops blend in 2 oz. carrier oil.

Ointment or unguent: For acute condition and topical use such as work on accupressure points and chakras, acute muscle or joint pain.
   50 drops blend in 1 oz. carrier oil.

Face oil: 10 drops blend in 1 oz. jojoba or carrier oil.

Bath gel, bath oil: 1/2 oz. blend in 12 oz. neutral gel or oil.

Lotion: 40 drops blend in 4 oz. neutral lotion.

Shampoo or conditioner: 50 drops blend in 4 oz. neutral shampoo or conditioner.

Hair oil: 50 drops blend in 2 oz. jojoba oil.

See also Chapter V (How to Use Essential Oils) for more detailed information on the different preparations.

The Carriers

Many vegetable oils can be used as carriers for aromatherapy preparations. Here some of the benefits of some of the most common carriers.

Apricot kernel oil: A fine and nourishing oil, especially recommended for skin care.

Avocado oil: Mostly used in skin care for its nourishing and restorative properties and its high vitamin content.

Borage oil: Very popular in Europe for skin care. It has one of the highest gammalinoleic acid (GLA) contents (19-24%). GLA is the origin of one class of protaglandin. It increases the protecting function of skin cells and reinforces the skin as a protecting membrane. Research has demonstrated that GLA applied to the skin is incorporated into the phospholipid molecules. Recommended in face oils for its rejunevative power. Should be kept refrigerated.

Canola: "Canadian oil," from rapeseed, an oil of antiquity recently rediscovered. It is very light and odorless, and penetrates easily, which makes it very good massage oil base. Its high linoleic acid content prevents rancidity.

Evening primrose: An expensive oil, rich in gamma-linoleic acid, therefore excellent for skin care (cf. borage oil). I recommend adding small amounts to a face oil. This oil, being highly unsaturated becomes ranid easily and should be kept refrigerated.

Grapeseed oil: A fairly new oil on the American market, this is becoming very popular among beauticians and massage therapists. Very light and odorless, it absorbs easily through the skin. Cleanser and toner.

Hazelnut oil: Moisturizing, nourishing, this oil has numerous uses in skin care preparations (cold creams, massage oils, body oils, lipsticks, etc.).

Jojoba oil: Jojoba oil is actually a wax, and therefore it does not become rancid, which makes it the ideal carrier for perfume oils. Some claim that it may have a tendency to clog the pores, while other authors find it very emollient and nourishing for the skin. It is also excellent for hair care (recommended for hair oil base).

Rosa musceta: From Chilean rosehip seeds. Another oil with high gammalinoleic acid content. It is emollient, nourishing, a tissue regenerator. Recommended for face oils.

Sesame oil: Sun protection. Sesamol and sesamoline are natural antioxidants (found only in the virgin cold-pressed oil).

Wheatgerm oil: Rich in vitamins E, A, and B. Its antioxidant properties make it useful in oilbase preparations to prevent rancidity. It helps regenerate tissues and promotes skin elasticity. Being rather heavy and having a fairly strong oder, it is used in small amounts in the carrier.

Suggested base for a face oil (3 oz. preparation):

Grapeseed: 1 oz.

Jojoba: 1 oz.

Wheatgerm: 1/2 oz.

Evening primrose, borage, or rosa musceta (or a combination of the three): 1/2 oz.

Suggested base for a massage oil (4 oz. preparation):

Canola oil: 2 oz.

Grapeseed oil: 1.5 oz.

Wheatgerm oil: 0.5 oz.

The Problem of Rancidity

Except for jojoba, which is a wax, any vegetable oil will eventually oxidize and become rancid. Keep your bases in closely covered, dark bottles and store them in a cool place (the refrigerator, if you do not use them often). I have noticed that essential oils have antioxidant properties; aromatherapy preparations will keep longer than the carriers alone. They have some shelf life, but still eventually go rancid. If stored properly, any oil-base preparation should keep for at least 6 months.

FORMULAS FOR SOME COMMON AILMENTS

Several manufacturers offer an extensive range of premixed blends for a wide range of indications (Aroma Vera, Inc., Ledet Oils, Original Swiss Aromatics; see resource guide).

I encourage you, however, to prepare your own blends. It really adds to the fun and the efficacy of your aromatherapy treatment. The following formulas will give you some guidelines. Once you become better acquainted with the power of the oils, you will be able to create your own blends.

Formulas for Accumulation/Elimination and Related Problems

Accumulation (toxins, fluids), elimination problems		Cellulitis		Obesity, water retention	
angelica root	5 %	fennel	10%	fennel	10%
caraway seeds	5 %	grapefruit	15%	grapefruit	25 %
carrot seed	5 %	thyme red	5 %	lemon	20 %
coriander seeds	5 %	cypress	10%	lime	10%
fennel	10%	birch	10%	orange	10%
juniper	10%	geranium	10%	tangerine	10%
birch	20%	lemon	20%	thyme, red	5 %
Grapefruit	20%	rosemary	20%	birch	10%
Orange	20%				

Application Methods: bath, compress, massage, friction/unguent, body wrap.

Complementary Treatment:
> Diet: drink a lot of liquids (herb teas or water), including one glass first thing in the morning. Cut down on meat, carbohydrates, milk products, salt. Eat a lot of raw or steamed vegetables (especially roots).
> Exercise.
> Cellulitis: massage, frictions, cold showers.
> Obesity: emotional support or psychotherapy might be necessary. Build up self-esteem. Be good to yourself.

Menstrual and Related Problems; Feminine Cycle

Amenorrhea, dismenorrhea		Feminine reproductive system (regulation)		Frigidity	
chamomile, mixta	10%	chamomile, Roman	5%	clary sage	5%
chamomile, Roman	5%	chamomile, German	5%	jasmine	10%
chamomile, German	5%	clary sage	5%	rose	10%
mugwort	10%	fennel	5%	ylang ylang	20%
pennyroyal	10%	rose	5%	sandalwood	10%
clary	5%	marjoram	40%	tangerine	45%
fennel	10%	lavender	35%		
marjoram	20%				
lavender	25%				

Menopause		Premenstrual syndrome	
chamomile, Roman	5%	clary sage	10%
chamomile, German	5%	fennel	10%
mugwort	5%	carrot seed	5%
sage	5%	lavender	20%
geranium	10%	marjoram	30%
bergamot	20%	mugwort	5%
lavender	25%	rosewood	20%
jasmine	5%		
ylang ylang	20%		

Application Methods: bath, compress, massage, friction/unguent, douche.

Articular and Muscular Problems

Arthritis		Muscular and articular pain		Rheumatism	
birch	30%	birch	40%	birch	20%
ginger root	10%	oregano	5%	cajeput	10%
juniper	10%	bay	5%	ginger root	10%
marjoram	20%	pepper	5%	juniper	10%
rosemary	20%	peppermint	20%	rosemary	10%

Arthritis		Muscular and articular pain		Rheumatism	
thyme, red	5%	clove buds	5%	thyme, red	5%
vetiver	5%	nutmeg	10%	marjoram	20%
		rosemary	10%	nutmeg	10%
				pepper	5%

Application Methods: bath, compress, massage, poultice, friction/unguent.

Complementary Treatment:
Diet: Drink a lot of liquids (herb tea and water). Cut down on salt. Eat raw and steamed vegetables (celery, cabbage, roots).
Massage and bath are particularly indicated.
Moderate exercise.

Respiratory-Related Disorders

Bronchitis		Colds		Respiratory system	
eucalyptus	30%	pine	20%	cajeput	20%
fir	20%	spruce	20%	eucalyptus	20%
hyssop	10%	therebentine	20%	fir	20%
lavender	10%	eucalyptus	20%	lavender	20%
myrtle	10%	lavender	20%	niaouli	10%
pine	10%			peppermint	10%
spruce	10%				

Respiratory weakness		Sinusitis	
fir	40%	eucalyptus	40%
pine	30%	lavender	40%
spruce	30%	peppermint	20%

Application Methods: diffuser, compress, massage, friction/unguent.

Complementary Treatment:
Breathing exercises, walks in forest or along beaches.
Diet: cut down on carbohydrates and milk products.

Blood Circulation and Digestion

Bruises		Circulation (varicosis, cold feet, tired legs)		Digestive system		Fatigue, anemia, convalescence	
everlasting	20%	benzoin resinoid	15%	bergamot	10%	basil	10%
geranium	20%	cinnamon leaf	5%	caraway seeds	5%	cardamom	10%
lavender	50%	cypress	20%	cardamom	5%	ginger root	10%
chamomile, blue	10%	lemon	30%	coriander seeds	5%	juniper	5%
		oregano	10%	fennel	5%	nutmeg	10%
		geranium	20%	ginger root	5%	peppermint	10%
				grapefruit	10%	rosemary	30%
				lemon	25%	spearmint	15%
				orange	20%		
				tangerine	20%		

Application Methods (Bruises): lotion, friction/unguent.

Application Methods (Circulation): bath, compress, massage, friction/unguent, body wrap.

Application Methods (Digestive system): bath, massage, friction/unguent.

Application Methods (Fatigue, anemia, convalescence): bath, diffuser, massage, friction/unguent.

Headaches, Impotence, Infectious Diseases

Headache		Migraines		Migraines (digestive origin)	
chamomile, Roman	10%	lavender	30%	basil	10%
peppermint	20%	marjoram	30%	chamomile, Roman	10%
rosewood	40%	melissa	10%	ginger root	10%
spearmint	10%	peppermint	20%	lavender	20%
lavender	20%	spearmint	10%	marjoram	30%
				peppermint	20%
				spearmint	10%

Application Methods: compress, diffuser, massage, friction/unguent.

Complementary Treatment:
Relaxation, breathing exercises.
Avoid heavy food (meat, eggs, rich sauces, etc).
Physical exercise.

Impotence (Oriental blend)		(Spicy blend)	
clary sage	10%	clary sage	10%
jasmine	20%	ginger root	10%
sandalwood, Mysore	20%	nutmeg	10%
ylang ylang	20%	pepper	10%
rosewood	20%	peppermint	10%
vetiver	10%	sandalwood, Mysore	20%
		ylang ylang	20%
		vetiver	10%

Application Methods: Bath, compress, massage, friction/unguent.

Complementary Treatment:

Relaxation, exercise. Avoid stress. Eat proteins and spicy, earthy food (meat may be recommended). Avoid alcohol excess.

Infectious diseases, epidemics (prevention)	
eucalyptus	30%
lavender	20%
myrtle	20%
peppermint	10%
tea tree	10%
thyme, red	10%

Application Methods: bath, compress, diffuser, massage, friction/unguent.

Insect Repellents

Fleas		Mosquitoes		Moths	
lavender	30%	citronella	25%	lavender	50%
lavandin	30%	geranium	25%	lavandin	50%
pennyroyal	20%	lemongrass	25%		
spike	20%	pennyroyal	25%		

Application Methods (fleas): diffuser, friction/unguent, sprinkle in infested areas.

Application Methods (mosquitoes): diffuser, lotion, friction/unguent.

Application Methods (moths): diffuser, aromatic pottery.

Insomnia

chamomile, Roman	10%	marjoram	20%
lavender	20%	neroli	20%
marjoram	20%	orange	20%
orange	20%	tangerine	20%
tangerine	20%	ylang ylang	20%
ylang ylang	10%		

<u>Application Methods:</u> bath, diffuser, massage.

<u>Complementary Treatment:</u>
Relaxation, yoga, breathing exercise.
Physical exercise (work out).
Avoid stress.
Balance your diet. Vitamins and minerals are advised.

Formulas for Emotional Problems, Stress, and Brain Stimulation

The blends in this section should be used in diffuser, massage, and bath.

Anxiety		Depression (indulging formula)		Depression (uplifting formula)	
benzoin resinoid	10%	bergamot	10%	lemon	10%
bergamot	10%	geranium	15%	lime	20%
clary sage	10%	jasmine	10%	melissa	10%
jasmine	10%	petitgrain	10%	peppermint	10%
lemon	10%	rose	5%	petitgrain	20%
patchouli	10%	sandalwood, Mysore	10%	rosemary	20%
petitgrain	20%	ylang ylang	20%	thyme, lemon	10%
rosewood	20%	rosewood	20%		

<u>Complementary Treatment:</u>
Relax, be good to yourself, treat yourself.
Start a new project. Physical exercise is strongly recommended.
Balance your diet. Vitamins and minerals are suggested.

Emotional shock, grief		Neurasthenia		Sadness	
melissa	10%	lavender	20%	benzoin resinoid	20%
neroli	10%	melissa	10%	rosewood	40%
rose	10%	patchouli	10%	jasmine	10%
tangerine	60%	rosemary	40%	rose	10%
sandalwood	10%	thyme, lemon	20%	ylang ylang	20%

Complementary Treatment:
Yoga, meditation. Psychotherapy and emotional support are strongly advised.

Energy		Memory (poor)		Mental fatigue	
benzoin resinoid	10%	basil	10%	basil	20%
cedarwood	20%	clove buds	10%	cardamom	20%
clary sage	10%	ginger root	10%	ginger root	20%
fir	30%	juniper	10%	peppermint	20%
spruce	30%	petitgrain	30%	rosemary	20%
		rosemary	30%		

Complementary Treatment:
Vitamins and minerals.
Reduce stress.
Balance diet (make sure to get enough proteins).

Nervous tension, nervousness		Stress		Tension	
geranium	10%	cedarwood	15%	clary sage	20%
lavender	10%	clary sage	10%	marjoram	20%
marjoram	20%	fir	20%	lavender	20%
melissa	10%	pine	15%	ylang ylang	20%
neroli	10%	spruce	20%	petitgrain	20%
tangerine	30%	ylang ylang	20%		
ylang ylang	10%				

Complementary Treatment:
Relaxation (yoga or meditation).
Massage and bath are strongly recommended.

Skin-Care Formulas

The following blends will be used in facials, masks, compresses, lotions, facial and body oils, and body wraps.

Acne		Dermatitis		Wrinkles	
bergamot	10%	cedarwood	10%	clary sage	5%
juniper	5%	juniper	5%	frankincense	5%
lavender	10%	lavender	10%	myrrh	5%
palmarosa	20%	*Litsea cubebaba*	10%	patchouli	5%
peppermint	5%	palmarosa	20%	rose	10%
rosemary	10%	peppermint	10%	rosemary	20%
sandalwood, Mysore	10%	rosewood	20%	rosewood	30%
thyme, lemon	30%	thyme, lemon	15%	geranium	20%

Dry skin		Oily skin		Sensitive skin	
clary sage	10%	clary sage	10%	chamomile, Roman	5%
jasmine	10%	ylang ylang	20%	everlasting	5%
palmarosa	30%	lavender	10%	jasmine	10%
rosemary	20%	lemon	30%	neroli	10%
rose	10%	geranium	20%	rose	10%
sandalwood	20%	frankincense	10%	rosewood	60%

Hair-Care Formulas

Use in shampoo, rinses, lotions, hair oils.

Oily hair		Hair loss, hair growth		Dandruff	
cedarwood	25%	bay	20%	cedarwood	20%
sage	25%	clary sage	10%	patchouli	20%
lemongrass	25%	ylang ylang	20%	rosemary	20%
rosemary	25%	cedarwood	20%	sage	20%
		rosemary	20%	tea tree	20%
		sage	10%		

Chakra, Energy Formulas

Use in unguent, diffuser, massage.

Crown chakra		Third eye		Heart chakra	
benzoin resinoid	10%	cistus	5%	benzoin resinoid	40%
cistus	5%	frankincense	5%	melissa	10%
frankincense	5%	myrrh	10%	neroli	30%
myrrh	10%	sandalwood, Mysore	20%	rose	20%
sandalwood, Mysore	20%	spruce	50%		
spruce	40%	mugwort	10%		
rose	10%				

Solar plexus		Sexual chakra		Root chakra	
rosemary	30%	jasmine	20%	pepper	40%
sage	20%	ylang ylang	30%	vetiver	30%
lemon	30%	sandalwood	20%	frankincense	30%
clove	10%	tangerine	30%		
juniper	10%				

Yoga, meditation, rituals		Astral body		Psychic centers	
cedarwood	20%	lavender	20%	cistus	5%
cistus	5%	marjoram	30%	elemi	10%
fir	30%	melissa	10%	frankincense	10%
myrrh	5%	patchouli	10%	myrrh	10%
sandalwood, Mysore	15%	rosemary	20%	cedarwood	25%
spruce	25%	thyme, lemon	10%	spruce	40%

NINE

Aromatherapy Reference Tables

The two following tables have been created to help you find rapidly the information that you may need in your daily practice. They might seem quite overwhelming at first glance. I hope you will find them comprehensive and practical at the same time.

Many oils are listed here that cannot easily be found in any other book. I also differentiate between the varieties of the same species (such as chamomiles, or the chemotypes of thyme). Considering that there are a few hundred essential oils, some have obviously been left out. Still, I cover here all the common oils plus all those that present some therapeutic interest and can be found on the market.

In the essential oils reference table, I give codes to show suggested uses of oils for the specific conditions.

In this coding system:
   D stands for diffuser
   M stands for massage
   B stands for bath
   F stands for facial masks
   C stands for compresses
   L stands for lotions
   O stands for face oil/body oil
   U stands for unguents

I also indicate the power of the oil with regard to the specific condition. I hope all this information will prove useful to the practitioner.

ESSENTIAL OILS REFERENCE TABLE

Oil Name	Property	Indication	Use	Power
angelica root	**Medicinal**			
Angelica	cleanser, depurative, drainer	accumulation (toxins, fluids)	MBFCLO	4
archangelica	stimulant digestive	digestive problems, migraine	DCU	3
Umbelliferae	revitalizing, stimulant	anemia, asthenia, anorexia, convalescence, rachitism	DMB	4
	carminative	aerophagia	MBC	3
	cleanser, depurative, drainer	gout	MCU	3
	antispasmodic	digestive spasms	MBCU	3
aniseed	**Medicinal**			
Pimpinella anisum	carminative	aerophagia	MBC	4
Umbelliferae	digestive stimulant	digestive problems, migraine	DCU	4
	antispasmodic	digestive spasms	MBCU	3
	galactagogue	insufficient milk	MBCU	3
	aphrodisiac	frigidity, impotence	MBCU	2
basil	**Medicinal**			
Ocymum basilicum	antiseptic (intestinal)	intestinal infections	MCU	3
Labiatae	stimulant	vital centers	DMBU	4
	cephalic	migraine	DCU	4
	antispasmodic, stomachic	dyspepsia, gastric spasms	MCU	3
	facilitates birth and nursing	nursing, pregnancy	DMBU	2
	Mind, emotion, psyche			
	stimulant	memory (poor), neurovegetative system	DMBU	4
	tonic (nervous)	nervous fatigue, intellectual, mental fatigue, mental strain	DMBU	4
	Contraindications			
	stupefying	high doses		2
bay	**Body care, skin care**			
Pimenta racemosa	scalp stimulant	hair growth	LO	4
Myrtaceae	**Medicinal**			
	antiseptic, stimulant	respiratory system	DMBCU	3
	antiseptic	infectious diseases	DMBCU	3
	analgesic, antineuralgic	pain (muscular and articular), neuralgia	MBCU	3

ESSENTIAL OILS REFERENCE TABLE (continued)

Oil Name	Property	Indication	Use	Power
Benzoin resinoid	**Body care, skin care**			
Styrax benzoin	rejuvenating, stimulant	skin elasticity	FCLOU	2
Styraceae	**Medicinal**			
	appeasing, balancing	energy inbalance	DMB	4
	regulator	secretions	MBCU	3
	expectorant	bronchitis	DMBC	3
	soothing	cough, laryngitis	D	3
	stimulant	circulation	MBCU	2
	antiseptic, diuretic	genitourinary infections, urinary infections	MBC	2
	healing	cracked and chapped skin, dermatitis, skin irritation, skin rashes, wounds	CLU	4
	Mind, emotion, psyche			
	purifier	drive out evil spirits	DU	3
	stimulant	crown chakra, heart chakra	DU	3
	comforting, euphoric	anxiety, loneliness, sadness	DMBU	3
	comforting, uplifting	exhaustion (psychic and emotional)	DMBU	3
bergamot	**Body care, skin care**			
Citrus bergamia	antiseptic, vulnerary	acne, eczema, seborrhea	FCLO	3
Rutaceae	**Medicinal uses**			
	refreshing	hot climates	DMBLU	3
	stimulant	digestive problems	MBC	3
	balancing	nervous system	DMBU	4
	antispasmodic, digestive	colics, intestinal infections	MCU	3
	antiseptic, vulnerary	leukorrhea, vaginal pruritus	MU	3
	Mind, emotion, psyche			
	antidepressant, uplifting	anxiety, depression	DMB	4
	Contraindications			
	increases photosensitivity	do not apply neat before sun	MFCLOU	3
birch	**Medicinal**			
Betula lenta &	analgesic	arthritis, pain (muscular and articular), rheumatism	MBCU	4
betula nigra				
Betulaceae	cleanser, depurative, drainer	accumulation (toxins, fluids),	MBCU	3

ESSENTIAL OILS REFERENCE TABLE (continued)

Oil Name	Property	Indication	Use	Power
		cellulitis, obesity, water retention		
	diuretic	cystitis, kidneys	MBCU	4
cajeput	**Medicinal**			
Melaleuca	balancing, reequilibrating	energy inbalance	DMB	3
leucadendron	antiseptic, antispasmodic	respiratory system	DMBCU	5
Myrtaceae	antiseptic	infectious diseases	DMBCU	4
	antiseptic (urinary)	cystitis, urethritis, urinary infections	MBC	4
	balsamic, expectorant	asthma, bronchitis, tuberculosis	DMBCU	5
	antineuralgic	rheumatism	MBCU	3
	antiseptic (intestinal)	amebas, diarrhea, dysentery	MB	3
	analgesic, antiseptic	earache	U	4
	antiseptic, expectorant	sinusitis	DU	5
caraway seeds,	**Medicinal**			
Carum carvi	cleanser, depurative, drainer	accumulation (toxins, fluids)	MBFCLO	3
Umbelliferae	stimulant, digestive stimulant	digestive problems	MBC	4
	stimulant general	energy deficiency	DMB	3
	carminative	aerophagia, fermentation	MBC	4
	antispasmodic	dyspepsia, migraine, digestive spasms	MBCU	3
	parasiticide	scabies	CLU	2
	diuretic	kidneys	MBCU	2
	tissue regenerator	infected wounds	FCLOU	3
	stimulant	glandular system	MBU	2
	Mind, emotion, psyche			
	tonic (nervous)	mental fatigue, mental strain	DMBU	3
cardamom,	**Medicinal**			
Eletteria	stimulant	digestive problems	MBC	4
cardamomum	aphrodisiac	impotence	MBCU	3
Zingiberaceae		diarrhea	MBCU	3
carrot seed	**Body care, skin care**			
Dauca carota	cleanser, depurative, drainer	dermatitis	MFCLOU	3
Umbelliferae	stimulate elasticity, tonic	aged skin, skin irritation, skin rashes, wrinkles	FCLO	3

ESSENTIAL OILS REFERENCE TABLE (continued)

Oil Name	Property	Indication	Use	Power
	Medicinal			
	cleanser, depurative, drainer	accumulation (toxins, fluids)	MBFCLO	4
	stimulant general	energy deficiency	DMB	2
	revitalizing, stimulant	anemia, asthenia, anorexia, convalescence, rachitism	DMB	3
	cleanser, depurative, hepatic	hepatobiliary disorders	MBCU	4
	emmenagogue	amenorrhea, dismennorrhea, premenstrual syndrome	MBCU	3
	stimulant	glandular system	MBU	3
chamomile, blue *Ormensis multicolis* Compositae	**Body care, skin care**			
	antiinflammatory, soothing	acne, dermatitis, eczema, skin care	FCLO	5
	antiinflammatory, soothing	inflamed skin, sensitive skin	FCLO	4
	Medicinal			
	analgesic, antiinflammatory	arthritis, inflamed joints	BCU	4
	antiinflammatory, healing, soothing	abscess, boils, bruises	CLU	4
	antispasmodic, sedative	colics, colitis	MCU	3
	cholagogue, hepatic	liver and spleen congestion	MCU	3
	analgesic, antiinflammatory	teething pain, toothache	U	3
chamomile, German *Chamomilla matricaria,* Compositae	**Body care, skin care**			
	antiinflammatory, soothing	acne, dermatitis, eczema, skin care	FCLO	3
	antiinflammatory, soothing	inflamed skin, sensitive skin	FCLO	4
	Medicinal			
	immunostimulant	leukocyte formation stimulant	DMU	4
	analgesic, antiinflammatory	arthritis, inflamed joint	BCU	4
	antiinflammatory, healing, soothing	abscess, boils	FCLO	4
	antispasmodic, sedative	colics, colitis	MCU	4
	calming, sedative	headache, insomnia, irritability, migraine	DCU	4
	emmenagogue	amenorrhea, dysmennorrhea, menopause	DMBCU	4
	analgesic	teething pain, toothache	U	4

ESSENTIAL OILS REFERENCE TABLE (continued)

Oil Name	Property	Indication	Use	Power
	antianemic	anemia, asthenia	DMB	4
	digestive, stomachic	digestive problems	MBC	4
	cholagogue, hepatic	liver, liver and spleen congestion	MCU	4
	balancing	feminine reproductive system	DMBCU	4
	Mind, emotion, psyche			
	appeasing	anger, tantrum	DMBU	4
chamomile, mixta	**Body care, skin care**			
	calming, soothing	sensitive skin	FCLO	4
Anthemis mixta,	**Medicinal**			
Compositae	antispasmodic, sedative	colic, colitis	MCU	3
	calming, sedative	headache, insomnia, irritability, migraine	DCU	3
	emmenagogue	amenorrhea, dysmennorrhea, menopause	DMBCU	3
	cholagogue, hepatic	liver and spleen congestion	MCU	3
chamomile, Roman	**Body care, skin care**			
	healing, soothing	abscess, boils, sensitive skin	FCLO	5
Anthemis nobilis	**Medicinal**			
Compositae	analgesic	arthritis, inflamed joint	BCU	3
	antispasmodic, sedative	colic, colitis	MCU	4
	calming, sedative	headache, insomnia, irritability, migraine	DCU	4
	emmenagogue	amenorrhea, dismennorrhea, menopause	DMBCU	4
	analgesic	teething pain, toothache	U	4
	antianemic	anemia, asthenia	DMB	4
	digestive, stomachic	digestive problems	MBC	4
	immunostimulant	leukocyte formation stimulant	DMU	4
	cholagogue, hepatic	liver, liver and spleen congestion	MCU	4
	balancing	feminine reproductive system	DMBCU	4
	Mind, emotion, psyche			
	realization	personal growth	DMBU	4
	appeasing	anger, oversensitivity, tantrum	DMBU	4

ESSENTIAL OILS REFERENCE TABLE (continued)

Oil Name	Property	Indication	Use	Power
cedarwood,	**Body care, skin care**			
Cedrus atlantica	antiseptic, fungicidal	dandruff, hair loss	LO	4
Confirae	antiseborrheic	oily hair	LO	3
	Medicinal			
	tonic	glandular system, nervous system, respiratory system	DMBCU	4
	antiseptic (urinary)	cystitis, urinary infections	MBC	3
	antiseptic, fungicidal	dermatitis, eczema, fungal infections, ulcers	FCLO	4
	Mind, emotion, psyche			
	appeasing	deep relaxation	DMBU	4
	appeasing, sedative	anxiety, stress	DMB	3
	elevating, grounding, opening	psychic work, yoga, meditation, rituals	DU	3
cinnamon bark	**Medicinal**			
Cinnamomum	stimulant	circulation, heart, nervous system	DMBU	4
zeylanicum				
Lauraceae	antiseptic	flu, infectious diseases	DMBCU	5
	antispasmodic	spasms	DMBC	2
	stimulant	anemia, asthenia, digestive problems	MBC	3
	parasiticide	lice, scabies	CLU	3
	aphrodisiac	impotence	MBCU	2
	antiseptic	intestinal infections	MCU	3
	contractions stimulant	childbirth	MCU	3
	Contraindications			
	irritant (skin)	high doses, neat or in high concentration	BFC	3
	convulsive	high doses		3
cinnamon leaf	**Medicinal**			
Cinnamomum	stimulant	circulation	MBCU	4
zeylanicum	antiseptic	infectious diseases	DMBCU	5
Lauraceae	parasiticide	lice, scabies	CLU	3
	antiseptic	intestinal infections	MCU	3
	Contraindications			
	irritant (skin)	high doses, neat or in high concentration	BFC	4
	convulsive	high doses		4

ESSENTIAL OILS REFERENCE TABLE (continued)

Oil Name	Property	Indication	Use	Power
cistus	**Medicinal**			
Cistus ladaniferus	diuretic	urinary infections	MBC	3
Cistaceae	drying, vulnerary	ulcers, wounds	CLU	2
	Mind, emotion, psyche			
	stimulant	third eye, crown chakra	DU	5
	stimulant	psychic centers	DU	5
	sedative (nervous)	insomnia, nervousness	DMBU	3
	elevating, grounding, opening	psychic work, yoga, meditation, rituals	DU	5
citronella	**Medicinal**			
Cymbopogon nardus	deodorant, deodorizer, purifier	sanitation, epidemics	D	4
Graminae	insect repellent	mosquitoes	DLU	5
	deodorant, deodorizer	bathroom, garbage	D	4
	stimulant	digestive problems	MBC	2
	antiseptic	infectious diseases	DMBCU	3
clary sage	**Body care, skin care**			
Salvia sclarea	cell regenerator	aged skin, wrinkles	FCLO	3
Labiatae	soothing	inflamed skin	FCLO	3
	regulator of seborrhea	dry skin, oily skin	FCLO	3
	regulator of seborrhea	oily hair	LO	3
	scalp stimulant, stimulant	hair growth	LO	3
	Medicinal			
	antispasmodic, emmenagogue	menstrual cramps, premenstrual syndrome	MBCU	4
	emmenagogue	amenorrhea, dysmennorhea	MBCU	4
	balancing, tonic	feminine reproductive system, feminine energy	DMBU	5
	Mind, emotion, psyche			
	antidepressant, calming	anxiety, emotional tension, stress, tension	DMBU	2
	antidepressant, euphoric	depression, postnatal depression	DMB	4
clove buds	**Medicinal**			
Eugenia	antiseptic, stimulant	respiratory system	DMBCU	5
caryophyllata	antiseptic	infectious diseases	DMBCU	4
Myrtaceae	antiseptic (urinary)	urinary infections	MBC	4

ESSENTIAL OILS REFERENCE TABLE (continued)

Oil Name	Property	Indication	Use	Power
	analgesic, antineuralgic	pain (muscular and articular), neuralgia, toothache	U	5
	carminative, stomachic	dyspepsia, fermentations	MBC	4
		anemia, asthenia, energy deficiency	DMB	4
	aphrodisiac	impotence	MBCU	3
	antiseptic, cicatrizant	infected wounds, ulcers	FCLO	3
	parasiticide	scabies	CLU	3
	Mind, emotion, psyche			
	stimulant (intellectual)	nervous fatigue, intellectual, memory (poor)	DMBU	4
coriander seeds	**Medicinal**			
Coriandrum	cleanser, depurative, drainer	accumulation (toxins, fluids)	MBFCLO	3
sativum	stimulant, digestive	digestive problems	MBC	4
Umbelliferae	revitalizing, stimulant	anemia, asthenia, convalescence	DMB	4
	carminative	aerophagia, flatulence	MBCU	4
	analgesic, warming	gout, rheumatism	MBCU	3
	aperitive, revitalizing	anorexia	DMB	3
	antispasmodic	migraine, digestive spasms	MBCU	3
	stimulant	glandular system	MBU	3
cumin seeds	**Medicinal**			
Cuminum	cleanser, depurative, drainer	accumulation (toxins, fluids)	MBFCLO	3
cymimum	revitalizing, stimulant	anemia, asthenia, convalescence	DMB	3
Umbelliferae				
	carminative	aerophagia, flatulence	MBCU	4
	antispasmodic	digestive spasms	MBCU	3
	digestive	digestive problems, migraine	DCU	3
	stimulant	heart, nervous system	DMBU	3
cypress,	**Medicinal**			
Cupressus	warming	energy deficiency	DMB	4
sempervirens	tonic	respiratory system	DMBCU	3
Coniferae	tonic (circulation)	cellulitis, circulation	MBCU	5
	astringent	edema, water retention	MBCU	5
	antispasmodic	asthma, cough, whooping cough	DMC	4
	antisudorific, deodorant, deodorizer	perspiration (especially of feet)	MBCLU	4

ESSENTIAL OILS REFERENCE TABLE (continued)

Oil Name	Property	Indication	Use	Power
elemi	**Medicinal**			
Canarium	cooling, drying, vulnerary	infected wounds	FCLOU	3
luzonicum	regulator	secretions	MBCU	4
Burseraceae	balsamic, expectorant	catarrhal condition	D	2
	balsamic	respiratory system	DMBCU	2
	Mind, emotion, psyche			
	fortifying	psychic centers	DU	3
Eucalyptus	**Medicinal**			
australiana	balancing, reequilibrating	energy inbalance	DMB	4
Eucalyptus	antiseptic, stimulant	respiratory system	DMBCU	5
polybractea	antiseptic	infectious diseases	DMBCU	4
Myrtaceae	antiseptic (urinary)	urinary infections	MBC	4
	balsamic, expectorant	asthma, bronchitis, tuberculosis	DMBCU	5
	antidiabetic	diabetes	MB	3
	antiseptic, expectorant	sinusitis	DU	5
Eucalyptus	**Medicinal**			
citriodora	antiseptic, bactericide	infectious diseases	DMBCU	3
Myrtaceae	deodorant, deodorizer, disinfectant	sanitation	D	3
Eucalyptus	**Medicinal**			
globulus	balancing, reequilibrating	energy inbalance	DMB	4
Myrtaceae	antiseptic, stimulant	respiratory system	DMBCU	5
	antiseptic	infectious diseases	DMBCU	4
	antiseptic (urinary)	urinary infections	MBC	4
	balsamic, expectorant	asthma, bronchitis, tuberculosis	DMBCU	5
	vermifuge	ascarides, oxyurids	MBCU	3
	antidiabetic	diabetes	MB	3
everlasting	**Body care, skin care**			
Helicrysum	antiinflammatory, soothing	acne, dermatitis, skin care	FCLO	3
italicum	antiinflammatory, soothing	inflamed skin, sensitive skin	FCLO	4
Compositae	antiinflammatory, astringent, healing	hemorrhage, skin irritation,	FCLOU	5

ESSENTIAL OILS REFERENCE TABLE (continued)

Oil Name	Property	Indication	Use	Power
	Medicinal			
	antiinflammatory, healing, soothing	abscess, boils	FCLO	4
	tissue stimulant	wounds, cuts	CLU	5
	cholagogue, hepatic	liver, liver and spleen congestion	MCU	4
fennel	**Body care, skin care**			
Foeniculum	cleanser, detoxifier	orange-peel skin	MBCU	5
vulgare	**Medicinal**			
Umbelliferae	cleanser, depurative, drainer	accumulation (toxins, fluids)	MBFCLO	5
	stimulant, stimulant digestive	digestive problems	MBC	4
	revitalizing, stimulant	anemia, asthenia, rachitism	DMB	4
	carminative	aerophagia, flatulence	MBCU	3
	antispasmodic	digestive spasms	MBCU	3
	cleanser, detoxifier	cellulitis, obesity, orange peel skin, water retention	MBCU	5
	regulator	amenorrhea, dysmennorrhea, feminine reproductive system, premenstrual syndrome	MBCU	4
	galactagogue	insufficient milk (nursing), nursing	DMBU	4
	stimulant	glandular system, glandular system (estrogen)	MBU	4
	Contraindications			
	toxic	young children (under 6)	MBU	2
fir	**Medicinal uses**			
Abies balsamea	warming	respiratory weakness	DMBU	4
Coniferae	tonic	glandular system, nervous system, respiratory system	DMBCU	4
	antiseptic (urinary)	genitourinary infections, urinary infections	MBC	3
	antiseptic, expectorant	asthma, bronchitis	DMBC	4
	Mind, emotion, psyche			
	elevating, grounding, opening	psychic work	DU	5

ESSENTIAL OILS REFERENCE TABLE (continued)

Oil Name	Property	Indication	Use	Power
	elevating, grounding, opening	third eye, crown chakra	DU	5
	appeasing, sedative	anxiety stress	DMB	5
	elevating, grounding, opening	yoga, meditation, rituals	DU	5
frankincense *Boswellia carteri* Burseraceae	**Body care, skin care** revitalizing, tonic **Medicinal**	aged skin, wrinkles	FCLO	4
	cooling, drying, vulnerary	infected wounds inflammations	FCLU	4
	regulator	secretions	MBCU	4
	balsamic, expectorant	asthma, catarrhal condition, cough	D	3
	antiseptic (pulmonary)	lungs	DCU	3
	Mind, emotion, psyche fortifying	mind, psychic centers	DU	5
	stimulant	third eye, crown chakra	DU	4
geranium, *Pelargonium graveolens* and *roseum,* Geraniaceae	**Body care, skin care** antiseptic, astringent, cell regenerator **Medicinal**	acne, aged skin, dermatitis, oily skin, skin care	FCLO	3
	astringent, hemostatic	bruises, hemorrhage	CLU	4
	antiseptic	infectious diseases	DMBCU	3
	antidiabetic	diabetes	MB	3
	diuretic	kidney stones, kidneys	MBCU	3
	adrenal cortex stimulant	cellulitis, adrenocortical glands, menopause	DMBCU	3
	insect repellent	mosquitoes	DLU	3
	astringent	sore throat, tonsillitis	U	3
	antiseptic, cytophilactic	burns, wounds	CLU	3
	Mind, emotion, psyche stimulant, uplifting	depression, nervous tension	DMBU	3
ginger root *Zingiber officinale* Zingiberaceae	**Medicinal** stimulant	digestive problems, memory (poor), neurovegetative system, vital centers	DMBU	4

ESSENTIAL OILS REFERENCE TABLE (continued)

Oil Name	Property	Indication	Use	Power
	stimulant	digestive problems	MBC	3
	cephalic	migraine	DCU	3
	antispasmodic, stomachic	dyspepsia, gastric spasms	MCU	3
	analgesic	arthritis, rheumatism	MBCU	3
	febrifuge	fever	MBCU	3
	carminative	aerophagia, flatulence	MBCU	3
	aphrodisiac	impotence	MBCU	3
		diarrhea	MBCU	3
	antiseptic, astringent	sore throat, tonsillitis	U	3
	Mind, emotion, psyche			
	stimulant	memory (poor)	DMBU	4
grapefruit	**Medicinal**			
Citrus paradisi	stimulant	digestive problems	MBC	3
Rutaceae	control of liquid processes	lymphatic system and secretions, secretions	MBCU	5
	drainer, lymphatic stimulant	cellulitis, obesity, water retention	MBCU	5
hyssop	**Medicinal**			
Hysopus officinalis	stimulant	respiratory system, vital centers	DMBU	4
Labiatae	antispasmodic, balsamic, expectorant	asthma, bronchitis, catarrhal condition, whooping cough	DMC	5
	antispasmodic, expectorant	whooping cough	DMC	5
	hypertensor	hypotentsion	DMCU	4
	digestive, stomachic	digestive problems, dyspepsia	MCU	3
	cicatrizant, vulnerary	dermatitis, eczema, wounds	CLU	2
jasmine	**Body care, skin care**			
Jasminum	moisturizer, soothing	dry skin, sensitive skin	FCLO	3
officinalis	healing, soothing	dermatitis	MFCLOU	3
Oleaceae	**Medicinal**			
	aphrodisiac	frigidity, impotence	MBCU	5
	Mind, emotion, psyche			
	stimulant	sexual chakra	DMBU	5
	antidepressant, euphoric	anxiety, lethargy, menopause, sadness	DMBU	5
	uplifting	lack of confidence	DMBU	4

ESSENTIAL OILS REFERENCE TABLE (continued)

Oil Name	Property	Indication	Use	Power
	antidepressant, euphoric	depression, postnatal depression	DMB	5
juniper *Juniperus communis* Coniferae	**Body care, skin care** cleanser, detoxifier, drainer **Medicinal**	acne, dermatitis, eczema	FCLO	4
	tonic	glandular system	MBU	4
	antiseptic (urinary)	genitourinary infections, urinary infections	MBC	5
	diuretic, urinary antiseptic	cystitis, diabetes, oliguria	MBCU	4
	cleanser, detoxifier, drainer	accumulation (toxins, fluids), arthritis, rheumatism, uric acid	MBCU	5
	Mind, emotion, psyche tonic (nervous)	nervous and intellectual fatigue, memory (poor)	DMBU	4
lavender *Lavandula officinalis* Labiatae	**Body care, skin care** antiseptic, cytophilactic	acne, dermatitis, eczema oily skin	FCLO	4
	healing **Medicinal**	psoriasis	CLU	3
	stimulant	metabolism, respiratory system, vital centers	DMBU	4
	antiseptic	blennorrhea, cystitis, infectious diseases	DMBCU	5
	antiseptic, cytophylactic	abscess, bruises, burns, wounds	CLU	5
	antiseptic, antispasmodic	asthma, bronchitis, catarrhal condition, colds	DMCU	4
	decongestant	sinusitis	DU	5
	calming, cephalic	headache, migraine	DCU	4
	calming	insomnia, nervous tension, palpitations	DMBC	3
	insect repellent	fleas, moth	DU	3
	antispasmodic, emmenagogue	amenorrhea, dismenorrhea, menopause, premenstrual syndrome	MBCU	3

ESSENTIAL OILS REFERENCE TABLE (continued)

Oil Name	Property	Indication	Use	Power
	Mind, emotion, psyche			
	appeasing	astral body	DMBU	4
	antidepressant, calming	depression, neurasthenia	DMB	4
	anticonvulsive	convulsions	DMBC	4
lavandin	**Medicinal**			
Lavandula fragrans	stimulant	respiratory system	DMBCU	3
delphinensis	antiseptic	infectious diseases	DMBCU	4
Labiatae	antiseptic, cythophilactic	burns, wounds	CLU	3
	deodorant, deodorizer, disinfectant	sanitation, epidemics	D	3
	insect repellent	fleas, mosquitoes	DLU	3
	Mind, emotion, psyche			
	appeasing	astral body	DMBU	3
lemon	**Body care, skin care**			
Citrus limonum	antiseptic, depurative, lymphatic stimulant	oily skin, skin care	FCLO	4
Rutaceae	**Medicinal**			
	digestive, stimulant	digestive problems	MBC	4
	control of liquid processes	lymphatic system and secretions, secretions	MBCU	4
	hepatobiliary stimulant	gall bladder congestion, liver	MCU	4
	tonic	nervous system	DMBU	4
	antiseptic, immunostimulant	infectious diseases, viral diseases	DMU	4
	immunostimulant	leukocyte formation stimulant	DMU	5
	stimulant, tonic, uplifting	anemia, asthenia, convalescence	DMB	4
	blood fluidifier, hypotensive	hypertension, hyperviscosity	MBU	4
	antivirus	herpes, immune system (low)	DMB	3
	drainer, lymphatic stimulant	cellulitis, obesity, water retention	MBCU	4
	Mind, emotion, psyche			
	antidepressant, uplifting	anxiety, depression	DMB	4
lemongrass	**Body care, skin care**			
Cymbopogon	astringent, tonic	open pores	FCLO	3
citratus	**Medicinal**			
Graminae	deodorant, deodorizer,	sanitation	D	3

ESSENTIAL OILS REFERENCE TABLE (continued)

Oil Name	Property	Indication	Use	Power
	disinfectant			
	insect repellent	mosquitoes	DLU	2
	stimulant	digestive problems	MBC	3
	digestive, stomachic	digestive problems	MBC	3
	regulator	parasympathic system	DMB	3
	antiseptic	infectious diseases	DMBCU	3
	Contraindications			
	irritant (skin)	neat or high concentrations	MBFCLOU	2
lime	**Medicinal**			
Citrus limetta	refreshing	hot climates	DMBLU	4
Rutaceae	digestive, stimulant	digestive problems	MBC	4
	control of liquid processes	lymphatic system and secretions, secretions	MBCU	3
	hepatobiliary stimulant	gall bladder congestion, liver	MCU	4
	tonic	nervous system	DMBU	4
	stimulant, tonic, uplifting	anemia, asthenia, convalescence	DMB	3
	drainer, lymphatic stimulant	obesity, water retention	MBCU	3
	antiseptic, antispasmodic	asthma, bronchitis, catarrhal condition	D	3
	Mind, emotion, psyche			
	antidepressant, uplifting	anxiety, depression	DMB	4
Litsea cubeba	**Body care, skin care**			
Graminae	healing, soothing	dermatitis	MFCLOU	3
	Medicinal			
	deodorant, deodorizer, disinfectant	sanitation, epidemics	D	3
	stimulant	digestive problems	MBC	3
lovage root	**Medicinal**			
Legusticum	cleanser, depurative, drainer	accumulation (toxins, fluids)	MBFCLO	3
levisticum	stimulant, digestive stimulant	digestive problems, intestines	MBC	3
Umbelliferae	stimulant	kidneys	MBCU	3
	revitalizing, stimulant	anemia, asthenia	DMB	3
	carminative	aerophagy, flatulence	MBCU	3
		gout, rheumatism	MBCU	2
	antispasmodic	digestive spasms	MBCU	2
	diuretic	cystitis, albuminuria	MBCU	4

ESSENTIAL OILS REFERENCE TABLE (continued)

Oil Name	Property	Indication	Use	Power
	emmenagogue	amenorrhea, dysmennorrhea	MBCU	3
	diuretic	edema, urine retention, water retention	MBCU	3
	diuretic	edema, water retention	MBCU	3
marjoram, Wild Spanish, *Thymus mastichina* Labiatae	**Medicinal**			
	calming	respiratory system	DMBCU	2
	antispasmodic	spasms digestive, spasms respiratory	DMCU	4
	analgesic, sedative	migraine	DCU	4
	analgesic, sedative	arthritis, rheumatism	MBCU	3
	Mind, emotion, psyche			
	calming, sedative	insomnia, nervous tension	DMBU	3
marjoram *Origanum marjorana* *marjorana hortensi* Labiatae	**Medicinal**			
	antispasmodic	digestive spasms, respiratory spasms	DMCU	4
	antispasmodic, emmenagogue	amenorrhea, dysmenorrhea, premenstrual syndrome	MBCU	3
	hypotensor, vasodilatator	hypertension	MBU	4
	analgesic, sedative	migraine	DCU	4
	analgesic, sedative	arthritis, rheumatism	MBCU	3
	antispasmodic, digestive	dyspepsia, flatulence	MBCU	2
	Mind, emotion, psyche			
	appeasing	astral body	DMBU	4
	calming, sedative	insomnia, nervous tension, tension	DMBU	4
melissa *Melissa officinalis* Labiatae	**Body care, skin care**			
	antiseptic, cythophilactic	acne, dermatitis, eczema	FCLO	3
	Medicinal			
	stimulant	metabolism, vital centers	DMBU	4
	antivirus	viral diseases	DMU	4
	calming, sedative	insomnia, migraine, nervous tension	DMBC	4
	Mind, emotion, psyche			
	appeasing	astral body	DMBU	4
	antidepressant, calming	depression, neurasthenia	DMB	5
	stimulant	heart chakra	DU	5

ESSENTIAL OILS REFERENCE TABLE (continued)

Oil Name	Property	Indication	Use	Power
	appeasing, soothing, uplifting	emotional shock, grief	DMBU	5
mugwort	**Medicinal**			
Artemisia vulgaris	emmenagogue	amenorrhea, dysmennorhea, menopause, premenstrual syndrome	MBCU	5
Compositae				
	analgesic	teething pain, toothache	U	4
	balancing	feminine reproductive system	DMBCU	5
	cholagogue	hepatobiliary disorders	MBCU	3
	vermifuge	ascaris, oxyurides	MMBU	3
	Mind, emotion, psyche			
	opening	dream, psychic work	DU	5
	Contraindications			
	abortive	pregnancy	DMBU	4
myrrh	**Body care, skin care**			
Commiphora	revitalizing, tonic	aged skin, wrinkles	FCLO	4
myrrha	**Medicinal**			
Burseraceae	cooling, drying	inflammations	FCLU	4
	regulator	secretions	MBCU	4
	balsamic, expectorant	asthma, catarrhal condition, cough	D	4
	antiseptic (pulmonary)	lungs	DUC	3
	cooling, drying, vulnerary	infected wounds	FCLOU	4
	fungicidal	thrush	Douche	4
	antiseptic, astringent	cough, mouth ulcers and inflammations, sore throat	U	4
	Mind, emotion, psyche			
	fortifying	mind, psychic centers	DU	5
	stimulant	third eye, crown chakra	DU	4
myrtle	**Medicinal**			
Myrtus communis	balancing, reequilibrating	energy inbalance	DMB	4
Myrtaceae	antiseptic, stimulant	respiratory system	DMBCU	5
	antiseptic	infectious diseases	DMBCU	4
	antiseptic (urinary)	urinary infections	MBC	4
	balsamic, expectorant	asthma, bronchitis, tuberculosis	DMBCU	5

ESSENTIAL OILS REFERENCE TABLE (continued)

Oil Name	Property	Indication	Use	Power
neroli	**Body care, skin care**			
Citrus vulgaris	soothing	sensitive skin	FCLO	5
Rutaceae	**Medicinal**			
	hypotensor, sedative	palpitations	DMBC	3
	Mind, emotion, psyche			
	sedative	hysteria, insomnia, nervous tension, nervousness	DMBU	5
	antidepressant, sedative	emotional shock, grief	DMBU	5
	stimulant	heart chakra	DU	5
niaouli	**Medicinal**			
Melaleuca	balancing, reequilibrating	energy inbalance	DMB	4
viridiflora	antiseptic, stimulant	respiratory system	DMBCU	5
Myrtaceae	antiseptic	infectious diseases	DMBCU	4
	antiseptic (urinary)	urinary infections	MBC	4
	balsamic, expectorant	asthma, bronchitis, tuberculosis	DMBCU	5
	tissue stimulant	acne, burns, wounds	CLU	4
	anticatarrhal	catarrhal condition	D	5
	antiseptic, expectorant	sinusitis	DU	5
nutmeg	**Medicinal**			
Myristica fragrans	stimulant	digestive problems	MBC	4
Myristaceae	analgesic	pain (muscular and articular), neuralgia, rheumatism	MBCU	3
	aphrodisiac	impotence	MBCU	3
	carminative	flatuence	MBCU	3
	antiseptic	intestines	MBC	3
	Mind, emotion, psyche			
	stimulant	nervous and intellectual fatigue	DMB	3
	Contraindications			
	stupefying, toxic	high doses		3
orange	**Medicinal**			
Citrus auranthium	digestive, stimulant	digestive problems	MBC	3
Rutaceae	control of liquid processes	lymphatic system and secretions, secretions	MBCU	2
	drainer, lymphatic stimulant	obesity, water retention	MBCU	3
	hypotensor, sedative	palpitations	DMBC	2

ESSENTIAL OILS REFERENCE TABLE (continued)

Oil Name	Property	Indication	Use	Power
	digestive, stimulant	digestive problems	MBC	3
	Mind, emotion, psyche			
	sedative	hysteria, insomnia, nervous tension	DMBU	3
oregano	**Medicinal**			
Origanum vulgare	stimulant	metabolism, respiratory system, vital centers	DMBU	4
Labiatae	stimulant	metabolism	DMBU	4
	stimulant	respiratory system	DMBCU	4
	antitoxic, antivirus	viral diseases	DMU	5
	antiseptic, cytophilactic	abscess, burns, wounds	CLU	3
	antiseptic, antispasmodic	asthma, bronchitis, catarrhal condition	D	3
	antiseptic, antitoxic	infectious diseases	DMBCU	3
	antiseptic	blennorrhea, cystitis	MBCU	3
	revulsive, rubefacient	circulation, pain (muscular and articular), circulation (capillary)	MBCLOU	4
	Contraindications			
	irritant (skin)	neat or high concentration	BFC	4
palmarosa	**Body care, skin care**			
Cymbopogon	antiseptic, cell regenerator	acne, dermatitis, skin care	FCLO	3
martini	antiseptic, cell regenerator stimulant	skin care, general skin care	FCLO	3
Graminae	moisturizer, soothing	dry skin	FCLO	3
	Medicinal uses			
	stimulant	digestive problems	MBC	3
patchouli	**Body care skin care**			
Pogostemon	antiphlogistic, regenerator	acne, dermatitis, eczema	FCLO	4
patchouli	tissue regenerator	aged skin, cracked and chapped skin, wrinkles	FCLO	4
Labiatae	fungicidal, tissue regenerator	impetigo	FCL	3
	regulator	seborrhea	FCLO	3
	decongestant	skin care	FCLO	3
	Medicinal			
	fungicidal	dandruff, fungal infections	CLU	4

ESSENTIAL OILS REFERENCE TABLE (continued)

Oil Name	Property	Indication	Use	Power
	Mind, emotion, psyche			
	appeasing	astral body	DMBU	4
	antidepressant, calming	anxiety, neurasthenia	DMB	4
pennyroyal	**Medicinal**			
Mentha pelugium	digestive, stomachic	dyspepsia, gastralgia, nausea vomiting	MCU	4
Labiatae				
	emmenagogue	amenorrhea, dysmenorrhea	MBCU	4
	insect repellent	fleas, mosquitoes	DLU	4
	Contraindications			
	abortive	pregnancy	DMBU	5
	toxic	high doses		3
pepper	**Medicinal**			
Piper nigrum	stimulant	digestive problems, nervous system	DMBU	3
Piperaceae				
	aphrodisiac	impotence	MBCU	3
	antitoxic	food poisoning	MU	3
	digestive, stomachic	dyspepsia	MCU	3
	analgesic, rubefacient	pain (muscular and articular), neuralgia, rheumatism	MBCU	3
	febrifuge	fever	MBCU	2
	Mind, emotion, psyche			
	stimulant	root chakra	MU	3
	comforting	ungroundedness	DMBU	3
peppermint	**Body care, skin care**			
Mentha piperita	cleanser, decongestant	acne, dermatitis	MFCLOU	4
Labiatae	**Medicinal**			
	stimulant	metabolism, nervous system, respiratory system, vital centers	DMBU	4
	antiseptic	infectious diseases	DMBCU	3
	antiseptic, antispasmodic	asthma, bronchitis, catarrhal condition	D	3
	decongestant	sinusitis	DU	4
	calming, cephalic	headache, migraine	DCU	4
	stimulant (nervous system)	fainting, vertigo	DC	4
	digestive, stomachic	dyspepsia, gastralgia, nausea, vomiting	MCU	5
	cholagogue, hepatic	hepatobiliary disorders	MBCU	4
	febrifuge	fever	MBCU	4
	aphrodisiac	impotence	MBCU	4

ESSENTIAL OILS REFERENCE TABLE (continued)

Oil Name	Property	Indication	Use	Power
	analgesic, antineuralgic	pain (muscular and articular), neuralgia	MBCU	4
	Mind, emotion, psyche			
	antidepressant, tonic	depression, neurasthenia	DMB	4
	stimulant (nervous system)	fatigue, mental fatigue, mental strain	DMBU	5
petitgrain biguarade *bitter orange leaves* Rutaceae	**Medicinal**			
	digestive, stimulant	digestive problems	MBC	3
	antispasmodic, digestive	dyspepsia, flatulence	MBCU	3
	Mind, emotion, psyche			
	clarifying, refreshing	confusion	DMBU	4
	antidepressant, uplifting	anxiety, depression	DMB	3
	stimulant, tonic	memory (poor), mental fatigue, mental strain, nervous system	DMBU	4
pine *Pinus sylvestris* Coniferae	**Medicinal**			
	warming	respiratory weakness	DMBU	3
	tonic	glandular system, nervous system, respiratory system	DMBCU	3
	antiseptic (urinary)	genitourinary infections, urinary infections	MBC	3
	expectorant, pectoral	colds, sore throat	U	4
	Mind, emotion, psyche			
	appeasing, sedative	anxiety, stress	DMB	3
rose *Rosa centifolia* and *damascena* Rosaceae	**Body care, skin care**			
	cell regenerator	aged skin, eczema, sensitive skin, wrinkles	FCLO	5
	moisturizer	dry skin	FCLO	4
	Medicinal			
	regulator	feminine reproductive system	DMBCU	4
	aphrodisiac	frigidity, impotence	MBCU	4
	astringent, hemostatic	hemorrhage	CLU	3
	Mind, emotion, psyche			
	stimulant	heart chakra	DU	5
	uplifting	emotional shock, grief	DMBU	5
	antidepressant, uplifting	depression, nervous tension, sadness	DMBU	5
rosemary *Rosmarinus officinalis* Labiatae	**Body care, skin care**			
	antiseptic, cytophilactic	acne, dermatitis, eczema	FCLO	4
	regulator of seborrhea	dry skin	FCLO	3
	rejunevating	aged skin, wrinkles	FCLO	4

ESSENTIAL OILS REFERENCE TABLE (continued)

Oil Name	Property	Indication	Use	Power
	regulator, scalp stimulant	dandruff, hair loss, oily hair	LO	4
	Medicinal			
	antiseptic, cytophilactic	abscess, burns, wounds	CLU	3
	antiseptic, antispasmodic	asthma, bronchitis, catarrhal condition	D	3
	stimulant	adrenocortial glands, metabolism, respiratory system, vital centers	DMBU	4
	tonic	anemia, asthenia, debility	DMB	4
	stimulant (hepatobiliary)	cholecystitis, cirrhosis, gall bladder congestion, hangover, jaundice	DMBCU	4
	cardiotonic	heart	DMBU	3
	analgesic, rubefacient	arthritis, pain (muscular and articular)	MCU	3
	Mind, emotion, psyche			
	appeasing	astral body	DMBU	4
	antidepressant, uplifting	depression, neurasthenia	DMB	4
	tonic (nervous)	memory (poor), mental fatigue, mental strain	DMBU	4
rosewood *Aniba roseaodora* Lauraceae	**Body care, skin care**			
	antiseptic, cell regenerator	acne, dermatitis, skin care	FCLO	5
	cell regenerator, regenerator	aged skin, sensitive skin, wrinkles	FCLO	5
	Medicinal			
	calming, cephalic	headache, nausea	DMCU	4
	Mind, emotion, psyche			
	antidepressant, uplifting	anxiety, sadness	DMBU	4
sage lavandulifolia *Salvia officinalis* Labiatae	**Body care, skin care**			
	depurative, healing	acne, dermatitis, eczema	FCLO	4
	regulator of seborrhea	dandruff, hair loss	LO	4
	Medicinal uses			
	stimulant	adrenocortical glands, metabolism, nervous system, vital centers	DMBU	4
	stimulant	metabolism	DMBU	4
	stimulant	nervous system	DMBU	4

ESSENTIAL OILS REFERENCE TABLE (continued)

Oil Name	Property	Indication	Use	Power
	stimulant	adrenocortical glands	MB	4
	tonic	anemia, asthenia, debility	DMB	4
	stimulant (hepato-biliary)	cholecystitis, jaundice	DMBCU	4
	hypertensor	hypotension	DMCU	4
	emmenagogue	amenorrhea, dismenorrhea, menopause, sterility	MBCU	4
	antisudorific	sweating (excessive)	MBCLU	4
	Mind, emotion, psyche			
	antidepressant, uplifting	depression, neurasthenia	DMB	4
	tonic (nervous)	fatigue, mental fatigue, mental strain	DMBU	4
	Contraindications			
	abortive, toxic	high doses		4
sandalwood, Mysore *Santalum album* Santalaceae	**Body care, skin care**			
	healing, moisturizer, soothing	acne, cracked and chapped skin, dry skin	FCLO	3
	Medicinal			
	antiseptic (urinary)	blennorrhea, cystitis, gonorrhea	LU	3
	Mind, emotion, psyche			
	elevating, grounding, opening	third eye, crown chakra	DU	4
	elevating, grounding, opening	yoga, meditation, rituals	DU	5
	antidepressant, euphoric	depression	DMB	3
savory *Satureia montana* Labiatae	**Medicinal**			
	stimulant	nervous system	DMBU	4
	antibiotic, antiseptic	infectious diseases	DMBCU	5
	tonic	anemia, asthenia, debility	DMB	4
	analgesic, rubefacient	arthritis, rheumatism	MBCU	4
	Contraindications			
	irritant (skin)	neat or high concentration	BFC	4
spearmint *Mentha viridis* Labiatae	**Body care, skin care**			
	cleanser, decongestant	acne, dermatitis	MFCLOU	3
	Medicinal			
	decongestant	sinusitis	DU	3

ESSENTIAL OILS REFERENCE TABLE (continued)

Oil Name	Property	Indication	Use	Power
	stimulant	metabolism, nervous system, respiratory system, vital centers	DMBU	3
	antiseptic, antispasmodic	asthma, bronchitis, catarrhal condition	D	3
	calming, cephalic	headache, migraine	DCU	3
	digestive, stomachic	dyspepsia, nausea, vomiting	MCU	4
	digestive, stomachic	dyspepsia, gastralgia	MCU	4
	cholagogue, hepatic	hepatobiliary disorders	MBCU	4
	febrifuge	fever	MBCU	2
	Mind, emotion, psyche			
	antidepressant, tonic	depression, neurasthenia	DMB	4
	stimulant (nervous sytem)	fatigue, mental fatigue, mental strain	DMBU	3
spike	**Medicinal**			
lavandula spica	stimulant	respiratory system	DMBCU	4
Labiatae	insect repellent	fleas	DU	4
	analgesic, rubefacient	pain (muscular and articular), sport preparation	MCU	4
	antiseptic, cytophilactic	abscess, burns, wounds	CLU	3
spruce	**Medicinal**			
Picea mariana	tonic	glandular system, nervous system, respiratory system	DMBCU	3
Coniferae	warming	respiratory weakness	DMBU	5
	antiseptic, expectorant	asthma, bronchitis	DMBC	4
	Mind, emotion, psyche			
	elevating, grounding, opening	psychic work	DU	5
	elevating, grounding, opening	third eye, crown chakra	DU	5
	appeasing, sedative	anxiety, stress	DMB	5
	elevating, grounding, opening	yoga, meditation, rituals	DU	5
tangerine	**Medicinal**			
Citrus reticulata	digestive, stimulant	digestive problems	MBC	3
Rutaceae	control of liquid processes	lymphatic system and secretions, secretions	MBCU	2

ESSENTIAL OILS REFERENCE TABLE (continued)

Oil Name	Property	Indication	Use	Power
	antispasmodic, digestive	dyspepsia, flatulence	MBCU	3
	drainer, lymphatic stimulant	obesity, water retention	MBCU	2
	Mind, emotion, psyche			
	sedative	hysteria, insomnia, nervous tension, nervousness	DMBU	3
	sedative, soothing	emotional shock, grief	DMBU	2
tarragon	**Medicinal**			
Artemisia dracunculus	antispasmodic, digestive	digestive and intestinal spasms, dyspepsia, hiccup	MCU	4
Compositae	carminative	aerophagia, fermentation	MBC	4
	vermifuge	ascarides, oxyurids	MBCU	3
tea tree	**Body care, skin care**			
Melaleuca alternifolia	cicatrizant, fungicidal, vulnerary	abscess, acne, herpes, pruritis, skin irritation, skin rashes	FCLOU	4
Myrtaceae	fungidical	dandruff, hair care	LO	4
	Medicinal uses			
	antiseptic, stimulant	respiratory system	DMBCU	5
	antiinfectious	infectious diseases	DMBCU	4
	antiseptic (urinary)	urinary infections	MBC	4
	balsamic, expectorant	asthma, bronchitis, tuberculosis	DMBCU	5
	fungicidal	athlete's foot, *Candida*, fungal infections, ringworm, vaginitis	CLOU	5
	antiinfectious	infected wounds, sores	CLOU	4
therebentine	**Medicinal**			
Pinus maritimus	tonic	glandular system, respiratory system	DMBCU	3
Coniferae	antiseptic (urinary)	genitourinary infections, urinary infections	MBC	4
	antiseptic, expectorant	asthma, bronchitis	DMBC	4
	expectorant, pectoral	colds, sore throat	U	4
	antiseptic, expectorant	asthma, bronchitis	DMBC	4

ESSENTIAL OILS REFERENCE TABLE (continued)

Oil Name	Property	Indication	Use	Power
thyme, citriodora, *thymus vulgaris* chem. *citriodora* Labiatae	**Medicinal**			
	stimulant	metabolism, nervous system, vital centers	DMBU	4
	antibiotic, antiseptic	infectious diseases	DMBCU	3
	antiseptic, cythophilactic	abscess, burns, wounds	CLU	3
	antiseptic, antispasmodic	asthma, bronchitis, catarrhal condition	D	3
	tonic	anemia, asthenia, debility	DMB	3
	Mind, emotion, psyche			
	appeasing	astral body	DMBU	4
	antidepressant, uplifting	depression, neurasthenia	DMB	4
thyme, lemon *Thymus hiemalis* Labiatae	**Body care, skin care**			
	healing, soothing	acne, dermatitis, eczema	FCLO	4
	Medicinal			
	stimulant	metabolism, vital centers	DMBU	4
	antibiotic, antiseptic	infectious diseases	DMBCU	3
	antiseptic, cythophilactic	abscess, burns, wounds	CLU	3
	calming	insomnia, palpitations	DMBC	3
	Mind, emotion, psyche			
	antidepressant, uplifting	depression, neurasthenia	DMB	3
thyme, red *Tymus zygis* Labiatae	**Medicinal**			
	stimulant	metabolism, vital centers	DMBU	4
	antibiotic, antiseptic	infectious diseases	DMBCU	5
	antiseptic (intestinal)	intestinal infections	MCU	5
	antiseptic (urinary)	blennorrhea, cystitis	MBCU	3
	tonic	anemia, asthenia, debility	DMB	3
	analgesic, rubefacient	arthritis, circulation (capillary), rheumatism, sport preparation	MCU	4
	stimulant circulation capillar	cellulitis, circulation, obesity,	MBCLOU	3
	stimulant, uplifting	depression, neurasthenia	DMB	3
	Contraindications			
	irritant (skin)	neat or high concentration	BFC	4

ESSENTIAL OILS REFERENCE TABLE (continued)

Oil Name	Property	Indication	Use	Power
verbena, lemon	**Medicinal**			
Lippia citriodora	hepatobiliary stimulant	liver	MCU	3
Verbenaceae	calming	tachycardia	DMBCU	3
	Mind, emotion, psyche			
	regulator	neurovegetative system	DMBU	3
	calming	nervousness	DMBU	3
vetiver	**Medicinal**			
Andropogon	rubefacient	arthritis	MBCU	4
muricatus	**Mind, emotion, psyche**			
Graminae	stimulant	root chakra	MU	4
	comforting	ungroundedness	DMBU	4
ylang ylang	**Body care, skin care**			
Unona	antiseborrheic	oily skin	FCLO	3
odorantissimum	scalp stimulant	hair growth	LO	3
Anonaceae	**Medicinal**			
	hypotensive	hyperpnea, hypertension, palpitations, tachycardia	DMBCU	4
	aphrodisiac	frigidity, impotence	MBCU	4
	Mind, emotion, psyche			
	antidepressant, euphoric	depression, menopause, stress	DMB	3
	sedative	insomnia, nervous tension	DMBU	3
	stimulant	sexual chakra	DMBU	3
	calming, euphoric	anger, fear, frustration	DMBU	3

AROMATHERAPY THERAPEUTIC INDEX

Beauty Care, Skin Care, Hair Care

Acne

Bergamot, blue chamomile, German chamomile, everlasting, geranium, juniper, lavender, melissa, niaouli, palmarosa, patchouli, peppermint, rosemary, rosewood, sage lavandulifolia, Mysore sandalwood, spearmint, tea tree, lemon thyme.

Application Methods: compress, facial, mask, lotion, face oil/body oil.

Aged Skin

Carrot seed, clary sage, frankincense, geranium, myrrh, patchouli, rose, rosemary, rosewood.

Application Methods: compress, facial, mask, lotion, face oil/ body oil, body wrap.

Cracked and Chapped Skin

Benzoin resinoid, patchouli, Mysore sandalwood.

Application Methods: compress, facial, mask, lotion, friction/unguent.

Dandruff

Cedarwood, patchouli, rosemary, sage lavandulifolia, tea tree.

Application Methods: lotion, hair oil, shampoo.

Dermatitis

Benzoin resinoid, blue chamomile, German chamomile, carrot seed, cedarwood, everlasting, geranium, jasmine enfleurage, juniper, lavender, *Litsea cubeba*, melissa, palmarosa, patchouli, peppermint, rosemary, rosewood, sage lavandulifolia, spearmint, lemon thyme.

Application Methods: compress, facial, mask, lotion, massage, face oil/body oil, friction/unguent.

Dry skin

Clary sage, jasmine enfleurage, palmarosa, rose, rosemary, Mysore sandalwood.

Application Methods: compress, facial, mask, lotion, face oil/ body oil.

Eczema

Bergamot, blue chamomile, German chamomile, cedarwood, juniper, lavender, melissa, patchouli, rose, rosemary, sage lavandulifolia, lemon thyme.

Application Methods: compress, facial, mask, lotion, face oil/body oil.

Hair Growth

Bay, clary sage, ylang ylang.

Application Methods: lotion, face oil/body oil, shampoo.

Hair Loss

Cedarwood, rosemary, sage lavandulifolia, ylang ylang.

Application Methods: lotion, face oil/body oil, shampoo.

Inflamed Skin

Blue chamomile, German chamomile, clary sage, everlasting.

Application Methods: compress, facial, mask, lotion, face oil/body oil, body warp.

Oily Hair

Cedarwood, clary sage, rosemary.

Application Methods: lotion, face oil/body oil, shampoo.

Oily Skin

Clary sage, geranium, lavender, lemon, ylang ylang.

Application Methods: compress, facial, mask, lotion, face oil/body oil.

Seborrhea

Bergamot, patchouli, sage.

Application Methods: compress, facial, mask, lotion, face oil/body oil, body wrap.

Sensitive Skin

Blue chamomile, chamomile mixta, Roman chamomile, German chamomile, everlasting, jasmine enfleurage, neroli, rose, rosewood.

Application Methods: compress, facial, mask, mask, lotion, face oil/body oil, body wrap.

Skin Care

Blue chamomile, German chamomile, everlasting, geranium, lemon, palmarosa, patchouli, rosewood.

Application Methods: compress, facial, mask, lotion, face oil/body oil, body wrap.

Skin Irritation, Skin Rashes

Benzoin resinoid, carrot seed, everlasting, tea tree.

Application Methods: compress, facial, mask, lotion, face oil/body oil, friction/unguent.

Wrinkles

Carrot seed, clary sage, frankincense, myrrh, patchouli, rose, rosemary, rosewood.

Application Methods: compress, facial, mask, lotion, face oil/body oil.

Medicinal Indications

Abscess

Blue chamomile, Roman chamomile, German chamomile, everlasting, lavender, oregano, rosemary, spike, tea tree, thyme citriodora, lemon thyme.

Application Methods: compress, facial, mask, lotion face oil/body oil.

Accumulation (Toxins, Fluids)

Angelica root, birch, caraway seeds, carrot seed, coriander seeds, cumin seeds, fennel, juniper, lovage root.

Application Methods: bath, compress, facials, mask, lotion, massage, face oil/body oil, body wrap.

Adrenocortical glands

Geranium, rosemary, sage lavandulifolia.

Application Methods: bath, massage.

Aerophagy

Angelica root, aniseed, caraway seeds, cardamom, coriander seeds, cumin seeds, fennel, ginger root, lovage root, tarragon.

Application Methods: bath, compress, massage.

Amenorrhea, Dysmennorrhea

Chamomile mixta, Roman chamomile, German chamomile, carrot seed, clary sage, fennel, lavender, lovage root, marjoram, mugwort, pennyroyal, sage lavandulifolia.

Application Methods: bath, compress, massage, friction/unguent, douche.

Anemia, Asthenia

Angelica root, romain chamomile, German chamomile, carrot seed, cinnamon bark, clove buds, coriander seeds, cumin seeds, fennel, lemon, lime, lovage root, petitgrain biguarade, rosemary, sage lavandulifolia, savory, thyme citriodora, red thyme.

Application Methods: bath, diffuser, massage.

Anorexia

Angelica root, carrot seed, coriander seeds.

Application Methods: bath, diffuser, massage.

Arthritis

Birch, blue chamomile, Romain chamomile, German chamomile, ginger root, juniper, marjoram, wild Spanish marjoram, rosemary, savory, red thyme, vetiver.

Application Methods: bath, compress, massage. friction/unguent, body wrap.

Asthma
Cajeput, cypress, Eucalyptus australiana, Eucalyptus globulus, fir, frankincense, hyssop, lavender, lime, myrrh, myrtle, niaouli, oregano, peppermint, rosemary, spearmint, spruce, tea tree, therebentine, thyme citriodora.
Application Methods: bath, compress, diffuser, massage, friction/unguent.

Blennorrhea
Lavender, oregano, Mysore sandalwood, red thyme.
Application Methods: bath, massage, friction/unguent.

Boils
Blue chamomile, Roman chamomile, German chamomile, everlasting.
Application Methods: compress, facials, mask, lotion, face oil/body oil.

Bronchitis
Benzoin resinoid, lime, myrtle, niaouli, oregano, peppermint, rosemary, spearmint, spruce, tea tree, therebentine, thyme citriodora.
Application Methods: bath, compress, diffuser, massage.

Bruises
Blue chamomile, geranium, lavender, everlasting.
Application Methods: compress, lotion, friction/unguent.

Burns
Geranium, lavender, lavandin, niaouli, oregano, rosemary, spike, thyme citriodora, lemon thyme.
Application Methods: compress, lotion, friction/unguent.

Candida
Tea tree.
Application Methods: compress, lotion, face oil/body oil, friction/unguent, douche.

Catarrhal Condition
Frankincense, hyssop, lavender, lime, myrrh, niaouli, oregano, peppermint, rosemary, spearmint, thyme citriodora.
Application Methods: diffuser.

Cellulitis
Angelica root, birch, cypress, fennel, geranium, grapefruit, lemon, red thyme.
Application Methods: bath, compress, massage, friction/unguent, body wrap.

Circulation
Cinnamon bark, cinnamon leaf, cypress, lemon, oregano, red thyme.
Application Methods: bath, compress, massage, friction/unguent, body wrap.

Circulation (Capillary)
Oregano, red thyme.
Application Methods: bath, compress, lotion, lotion, massage, face oil/body oil, friction/unguent, body wrap.

Colds
Eucalyptus globulus, lavender, pine, spruce, therebentine.
Application Methods: compress, diffuser, massage, friction/unguent.

Convalescence
Angelica root, carrot seed, coriander seeds, cumin seeds, lemon, lime, petitgrain biguarade.
Application Methods: bath diffuser, massage.

Cough
Benzoin resinoid, cypress, frankincense, myrrh.
Application Methods: diffuser.

Cystitis
Birch, cajeput, cedarwood, juniper, lavender, lovage root, oregano, Mysore sandalwood, red thyme.

Application Methods: bath, compress, massage, friction/unguent.

Debility
Rosemary, sage lavandulifolia, savory, thyme citriodora, red thyme.
Application Methods: bath, diffuser, massage.

Diabetes
Eucalyptus australiana, Eucalyptus globulus, geranium, juniper.
Application Methods: bath, massage.

Digestive Problems
Angelica root, aniseed, bergamot, Roman chamomile, German chamomile, caraway seeds, cardamom, cinnamon bark, coriander seeds, cumin seeds, fennel ginger root, grapefruit, lemon, lemongrass, lime, *Litsea cubeba*, lovage root.
Application Methods: bath, compress, massage.

Dyspepsia
Basil, caraway seeds, clove buds, ginger root, hyssop, pennyroyal, pepper, peppermint, petitgrain biguarade, spearmint, tangerine, tarragon.
Application Methods: compress, massage, friction/ unguent.

Energy Deficiency
Caraway seeds, clove buds, cypress.
Application Methods: bath, diffuser, massage.

Energy Imbalance
Benzoin resinoid, cajeput, *Eucalyptus australiana, Eucalyptus globulus,* myrtle, niaouli.
Application Methods: bath, diffuser, massage.

Fainting
Peppermint.
Application Methods: compress, diffuser.

Feminine Reproductive System
Roman chamomile, German chamomile, clary sage, fennel, mugwort, rose.
Application Methods: bath, compress, diffuser, massage, friction/unguent, douche.

Fermentations
Caraway seeds, clove buds, tarragon.
Application Methods: bath, compress, massage.

Fever
Ginger root, peppermint.
Application Methods: bath, compress, massage, friction/unguent.

Flatulence
Cardamom, coriander seeds, cumin seeds, fennel, ginger root, lovage root, nutmeg, petitgrain biguarade, tangerine.
Application Methods: bath, compress, massage, friction/unguent.

Fleas
Lavender, lavandin, pennyroyal, spike.
Application Methods: diffuser, friction/unguent.

Frigidity
Clary sage, jasmine enfleurage, rose, ylang ylang.
Application Methods: bath, compress, diffuser, massage, friction/unguent.

Fungal Infections
Cedarwood, patchouli, tea tree.
Application Methods: compress, lotion, friction/ unguent, douche.

Gallbladder Congestion
Lemon, lime, rosemary.
Application Methods: bath, compress, massage, friction/unguent.

Gastric Spasms
Basil, ginger root, tarragon.
Application Methods: compress, massage, friction/ unguent.

Genitourinary Infections

Fir, juniper, pine, therebentine.
Application Methods: bath, compress, lotion, massage.

Glandular System

Carrot seed, cedarwood, coriander seeds, fennel, fir, juniper, pine, spruce, therebentine.
Application Methods: bath, massage, friction/unguent.

Gout

Angelica root, coriander seeds.
Application Methods: compress, massage, friction/unguent.

Headache

Chamomile mixta, Roman chamomile, German chamomile, lavender, peppermint, rosewood, spearmint.
Application Methods: bath, compress, diffusor, massage, friction/unguent.

Hemorrhage

Everlasting, geranium, rose.
Application Methods: compress, lotion, friction/unguent.

Hemorrhoids

Cypress.
Application Methods: compress, lotion, friction/unguent.

Hepatobiliary Disorders

Carrot seed, mugwort, pennyroyal, peppermint, spearmint.
Application Methods: bath, compress, massage, friction/unguent.

Herpes

Lemon, tea tree.
Application Methods: compress, face oil/body oil, friction/unguent.

Hiccup

Tarragon.
Application Methods: compress, massage, friction/unguent.

Hypertension

Lemon, marjoram, ylang ylang.
Application Methods: bath, massage, friction/unguent.

Hypotension

Hyssop, sage lavandulifolia.
Application Methods: compress, diffuser, massage, friction/unguent.

Immune System (Low)

Lemon, tea tree.
Application Methods: bath, diffuser, massage.

Impotence

Cardamom, clary sage, clove buds, ginger root, jasmine enfleurage, nutmeg, pepper, peppermint, rose, Mysore sandalwood, ylang ylang.
Application Methods: bath, compress, massage, friction/unguent.

Infectious Diseases

Bay, cajeput, cinnamon bark, cinnamon leaf, citronella, clove buds, *Eucalyptus australiana, Eucalyptus citriodora, Eucalyptus globulus,* geranium, lavender, lavandin, lemon, lemongrass, *Litsea cubeba,* myrtle, niaouli, oregano, peppermint, savory, tea tree, red thyme.
Application Methods: bath, compress, diffuser, massage, friction/unguent.

Inflamed Joint

Blue chamomile, German chamomile, Roman chamomile.
Application Methods: bath, compress, friction/unguent.

Inflammations

Frankincense, myrrh.

Application Methods: compress, facials, mask, lotion, friction/unguent.

Insomnia
Chamomile mixta, Roman chamomile, German chamomile, cistus, lavender, marjoram, wild Spanish marjoram, melissa, neroli, orange, tangerine, lemon thyme, ylang ylang.
Application Methods: bath, diffuser, massage, friction/unguent.

Insufficient Milk (Nursing)
Fennel.
Application Methods: compress, massage, friction/unguent.

Intestinal Infections
Basil, bergamot, cinnamon bark, cinnamon leaf, red thyme.
Application Methods: compress, massage, friction/unguent.

Intestines
Lovage root, nutmeg.
Application Methods: bath, compress, massage.

Kidneys
Birch, geranium, lovage root.
Application Methods: bath, compress, massage, friction/unguent.

Liver
Blue chamomile, chamomile mixta, German chamomile, Roman chamomile, everlasting.
Application Methods: compress, massage, friction/unguent.

Liver and Spleen Congestion
German chamomile, Roman chamomile, everlasting, lemon, lemon verbena, lime.
Application Methods: compress, massage, friction/unguent.

Lymphatic System and Secretions
Grapefruit, lemon, lime.
Application Methods: bath, massage, friction/unguent.

Menopause
Chamomile mixta, Roman chamomile, German chamomile, geranium, jasmine enfleurage, lavender, mugwort, sage lavandulifolia, ylang ylang.
Application Methods: bath, compress, diffuser, massage, friction/unguent.

Metabolism
Lavender, melissa, oregano, peppermint, rosemary, sage lavandulifolia, spearmint, thyme citriodora, lemon thyme, red thyme.
Application Methods: bath, diffuser, massage, friction/unguent.

Migraine
Angelica root, aniseed, basil, chamomile mixta, Roman chamomile, German chamomile, caraway seeds, coriander seeds, cumin seeds, ginger root, lavender, marjoram, wild Spanish marjoram, melissa, peppermint, spearmint.
Application Methods: compress, diffuser, friction/unguent.

Mosquitoes
Citronella, geranium, lavandin, pennyroyal.
Application Methods: diffuser, lotion, friction/unguent.

Moths
Lavender, lavandin.
Application Methods: diffuser, friction/unguent.

Nausea
Peppermint, rosewood, spearmint.
Application Methods: compress, diffuser, massage, friction/unguent.

Neuralgia
Bay, clove buds, nutmeg, pepper, peppermint.

Application Methods: bath, compress, massage, friction/unguent.

Obesity
Angelica root, birch, fennel, grapefruit, lemon, lime, orange, red thyme.
Application Methods: bath, compress, massage, friction/unguent, body wrap.

Pain (Muscular and Articular)
Bay, birch, clove buds, nutmeg, oregano, pepper, peppermint, rosemary, spike.
Application Methods: bath, compress, massage, friction/unguent.

Palpitations
Lavender, melissa, neroli, lemon thyme, ylang ylang.
Application Methods: bath, compress, diffuser, massage.

Perspiration (Especially Feet)
Cypress, sage.
Application Methods: bath, compress, lotion, massage, friction/unguent.

Premenstrual Syndrome
Carrot seed, clary sage, fennel, lavender, marjoram, mugwort.
Application Methods: bath, compress, massage, friction/unguent, douche.

Respiratory System
Bay, cajeput, cedarwood, clove buds, cypress, *Eucalyptus australiana, Eucalyptus globulus*, fir, hyssop, lavender, lavandin, myrtle, niaouli, oregano, peppermint, pine, rosemary, spearmint, spike, spruce, tea tree, therebentine.
Application Methods: bath, compress, diffuser, massage, friction/unguent.

Respiratory Weakness
Fir, pine, spruce.
Application Methods: bath, diffuser, massage, friction/unguent.

Rheumatism
Birch, cajeput, coriander seeds, ginger root, juniper, marjoram, wild Spanish marjoram, nutmeg, pepper, rosemary, savory, red thyme.
Application Methods: bath, compress, massage, friction/unguent.

Sanitation
Citronella, *Eucalyptus citriodora*, lavandin, lemongrass, litsea cubeda.
Application Methods: diffuser.

Secretions
Benzoin resinoid, elemi, frankincense, grapefruit, lemon, lime, myrrh.
Application Methods: bath, compress, massage, friction/unguent.

Sinusitis
Cajeput, *Eucalyptus australiana, Eucalyptus globulus*, lavender, myrtle, niaouli, peppermint, spearmint.
Application Methods: diffuser, friction/unguent.

Sore Throat
Geranium, ginger root, myrrh, pine, spruce, therebentine.
Application Methods: friction/unguent, gargle.

Spasms, Digestive
Angelica root, aniseed, caraway seeds, coriander seeds, cumin seeds, fennel, marjoram, wild Spanish marjoram.
Application Methods: bath, compress, massage, friction/unguent.

Tachycardia
Lemon verbena, ylang ylang.
Application Methods: bath, compress, diffuser, massage, friction/unguent.

Teething Pain
Blue chamomile, German chamomile, Roman chamomile, mugwort.
Application Methods: friction/unguent, gargle.

Tonsillitis
Geranium, ginger root, blue chamomile.
<u>Application Methods:</u> friction/unguent, gargle.

Toothache
Blue chamomile, German chamomile, Roman chamomile, clove buds, mugwort.
<u>Application Methods:</u> friction/unguent, gargle.

Tuberculosis
Cajeput, *Eucalyptus australiana, Eucalyptus globulus*, myrtle, niaouli, tea tree.
<u>Application Methods:</u> bath, compress, diffuser, massage, friction/unguent.

Urinary Infections
Cajeput, cedarwood, cistus, clove buds, *Eucalyptus australiana, Eucalyptus globulus*, fir, juniper, myrtle, niaouli, pine, tea tree, therebentine.
<u>Application Methods:</u> bath, compress, massage.

Varicosis
Cypress, lemon.
<u>Application Methods:</u> compress, lotion, friction/unguent.

Viral Diseases
Lemon, melissa, oregano.
<u>Application Methods:</u> Diffuser, massage, friction/unguent.

Vital Centers
Basil, ginger root, hyssop, lavender, melissa, oregano, peppermint, rosemary, sage lavandulifolia, spearmint, thyme citriodora, lemon thyme, red thyme.
<u>Application Methods:</u> bath, diffuser, massage, friction/unguent.

Vomiting
Peppermint, spearmint.
<u>Application Methods:</u> compress, massage, friction/unguent.

Water Retention
Angelica root, birch, cypress, fennel, grapefruit, lemon, lime, lovage root, orange.
<u>Application Methods:</u> bath, compress, massage, friction/unguent, body wrap.

Whooping Cough
Cypress, hyssop.
<u>Application Methods:</u> compress, diffuser, massage.

Wounds
Benzoin resinoid, everlasting, geranium, lavender, lavandin, niaouli, oregano, rosemary, spike, thyme citriodora, lemon thyme.
<u>Application Methods:</u> compress, lotion, friction/unguent.

Wounds (Infected)
Caraway seeds, clove buds, elemi, frankincense, myrrh, tea tree.
<u>Application Methods:</u> compress, facials, lotion, face oil/body oil, friction/unguent.

Mind, Emotions, Psyche

Anger
German chamomile, Roman chamomile, ylang ylang.
<u>Application Methods:</u> bath, diffuser, massage friction/unguent.

Anxiety
Benzoin resinoid, bergamot, cedarwood, fir, jasmine enfleurage, lemon, lime, pathchouli, petitgrain biguarade, pine, rosewood, spruce.
<u>Application Methods:</u> bath, diffuser, massage, friction/unguent.

Astral Body
Lavender, lavandin, marjoram, melissa, patchouli, rosemary, thyme citriodora.
<u>Application Methods:</u> bath, diffuser, massage, friction/unguent.

Confidence (Lack of)
Jasmine enfleurage.
Application Methods: bath, diffuser, massage, friction/unguent.

Confusion
Petitgrain biguarade.
Application Methods: bath, diffuser, massage, friction/unguent.

Depression
Bergamot, clary sage, geranium, jasmine enfleurage, lavender, lemon, lime, melissa, peppermint, petitgain biguarade, rose, rosemary, sage lavandulifolia, Mysore sandlwood, spearmint, thyme citriodora, lemon thyme, red thyme, ylang ylang.
Application Methods: bath, diffuser, massage.

Depression (Postnatal)
Clary sage, jasmine enfleurage.
Application Methods: bath, diffuser, massage.

Dream
Mugwort, clary sage.
Application Methods: diffuser, friction/unguent.

Emotional Shock
Melissa, neroli, rose.
Application Methods: bath, diffuser, massage, friction/unguent.

Fatigue, Nervous, Intellectual
Basil, clove buds, juniper, nutmeg.
Application Methods: bath, diffuser, massage.

Grief
Melissa, neroli, rose.
Application Methods: bath, diffuser, massage, friction/unguent.

Hysteria
Neroli, orange, tangerine.
Application Methods: bath, diffuser, massage.

Memory (Poor)
Basil, clove buds, ginger root, juniper, petitgrain biguarade, rosemary.
Application Methods: bath, diffuser, massage, friction/unguent.

Mental Fatigue, Mental Strain
Basil, caraway seeds, ginger root, peppermint, petitgrain biguarade, rosemary, sage lavandulifolia, spearmint.
Application Methods: bath, diffuser, massage, friction/unguent.

Mind
Frankincense, myrrh.
Application Methods: bath, diffuser, massage, friction/unguent.

Nervous System
Bergamot, cedarwood, cinnamon bark, cumin seeds, fir, lemon, lime, pepper, peppermint, petitgrain biguarade, pine, sage lavandulifolia, savory, spearmint, spruce, thyme citriodora.
Application Methods: bath, diffuser, massage, friction/unguent.

Nervous Tension
Geranium, lavender, marjoram, wild Spanish marjoram, melissa, neroli, orange, rose, tangerine, ylang ylang.
Application Methods: bath, diffuser, massage friction/unguent.

Nervousness
Cistus, neroli, orange, tangerine, lemon verbena.
Application Methods: bath, diffuser, massage friction/unuguent.

Neurasthenia
Lavender, melissa, patchouli, peppermint, rosemary, sage lavandulifolia, spearmint, thyme citriodora, lemon thyme, red thyme.
Application Methods: bath, diffuser, masssage.

Neurovegetative System
Basil, ginger root, lemon verbena.
Application Methods: bath, diffuser, massage, friction/unguent.

Psychic Centers
Cistus, elemi, frankincense, myrrh.
Application Methods: diffuser, friction/unguent.

Psychic Work
Cedarwood, cistus, mugwort, spruce.
Application Methods: diffuser, friction/unguent.

Sadness
Benzoin resinoid, jasmine enfleurage, rose, rosewood.
Application Methods: bath, diffuser, massage, friction/unguent.

Stress
Cedarwood, fir, pine, spruce, ylang ylang.
Application Methods: bath, diffuser, massage.

Tantrum
German chamomile, Roman chamomile.
Application Methods: bath, diffuser, massage, friction/unguent.

Ungroundedness
Pepper, vetiver.
Application Methods: bath, diffuser, massage, friction/unguent.

Yoga, Meditation, Rituals
Cedarwood, cistus, Mysore sandalwood, spruce.
Application Methods: diffuser, friction/unguent.

Chakras, Energy Centers

Crown Chakra
Benzoin resinoid, cistus, frankincense, myrrh, Mysore sandalwood, spruce.
Application Methods: diffuser, friction/unguent.

Heart Chakra
Benzoin resinoid, melissa, neroli, rose.
Application Methods: diffuser, friction/unguent.

Root Chakra
Pepper, vetiver.
Application Methods: massage, friction/unguent.

Sexual Chakra
Jasmine enfleurage, ylang ylang.
Application Methods: bath, diffuser, massage friction/unguent.

Third Eye
Cistus, frankincense, myrrh, Mysore sandalwood, spruce.
Application Methods: diffuser, friction/unguent.

Selected Bibliography

Fabrice Bardeau. *La medecine par les fleurs.* 1976.

P. Belaiche, M. Girault. *Traite de phystotherapie et d'aromatherapie,* 3 vols. Maloine Editeur, Paris, 1979. Extensive clinical data. P. Belaiche teaches aromatherapy in French medical schools.

The Holy Bible.

Hieronymus Braunschweig. *The vertuose boke of distyllacyon of the waters of all maner of herbes.* 1527.

Scott Cunningham. *Magical Aromatherapy.* Llewellyn Publications, St. Paul, MN, 1990. Scott explores different avenues for the uses of essential oils. Comprehensive, well written.

Patricia Davis. *Aromatherapy: An A-Z.* C. W. Daniel Company, Saffron Walden, Essex, United Kingdom, 1988. Patricia Davis founded the London School of Aromatherapy.

R. M. Gattefosse. *Aromatherapy.* Girardot Editeur, Paris, 1928. By the one who first coined the term "aromatherapy."

Judith Jackson. *Scentual Touch.* Henry Holt and Co., New York, 1986.

H. Leclerc. *Precis de phytotherapie.* Masson Editeur, Paris, 1954.

Nicholas Lemery. *Dictionaire des drogues simples.* 1759.

Marguerite Maury. *The Secret of Life and Youth.* 1961. Once a collector's item, now available as *Mme. Maury Guide to Aromatherapy.* C. W. Daniel Company, Saffron Walden, Essex, United Kingdom, 1988.

Joseph E. Mayer. *The Herbalist.* 1907.

Shirley Price. *Practical Aromatherapy.* Thorsons Publishing Group, Wellingborough, Northamptonshire, United Kingdom, 1983.

Danielle Ryman. *The Aromatherapy Handbook.* C.W. Daniel Company, Saffron Walden, Essex, England, 1984.

Robert Tisserand. *Aromatherapy to Heal and Tend the Body.* Lotus Light, Wilmot, WI, 1989. The new Tisserand. Some interesting case studies.

Robert Tisserand. *The Art of Aromatherapy.* Healing Arts Press, Rochester, VT, 1977. The British classic.

Jean Valnet. *The Practice of Aromatherapy.* Destiny Books, Rochester, VT, 1982. Still a classic, by the man who launched the revival of aromatherapy in France.

J. Valnet, C. Durrafour, J. C. Lappraz. *Phytotherapie et aromatherapie une medecine nouvelle.* Presses de la Renaissance, Paris, 1979. Dr. Durrafour and Dr. Lappraz also teach aromatherapy in France and Switzerland.

Valerie Worwood. *Aromantics.* Pan Books Ltd., London, 1987. Funny, well written, provocative. Certainly a different perspective.

Anthroposophy

Goethe. *Metamorphose des Plantes.* Editions Triades, Paris.

Dietrich Gumbel. *Principles of holistic skin therapy with herbal essences.* Karl F. Haug Publishers, Heidelberg, RFA, 1986.

Wilhelm Pelikan. *Heilpflanzenkunde*, 2 vols. Editions Triades, Paris, 1962. Absolutely fascinating. The author explains in great detail the energy aspect of medicinal plants and the botanical family approach. Available only in German edition and its French translation.

Essential Oils (Production)

Steffen Arctander. *Perfume and Flavor Materials of Natural Origin.* Published by the author, 6665 Valley View Blvd, Las Vegas, NV 89118, 1960.

E. Guenther. *The Essential Oils*, 4 vols., 1948-1952. Forty years later, still the bible. For serious readers only (over 10,000 pages).

Brian Lawrence. *Essential Oils*, 3 vols., 1976-1978, 1979-1980, 1981-1987. Allured Publishing Corporation, PO Box 318, Wheaton, IL 60189-0318. Reprints from Dr. Lawrence's columns in *Perfumer & Flavorist.* If the Guenther is the bible, the Lawrence could become the New Testament. For experts only.

Perfumery, Cosmetics, Fragrances

R. M. Gattefosse, H. Jonquieres. *Techniques of Beauty Products.* 1949.

Roy Genders. *A History of Scents.* 1972.

Boyd Gibbon. "The Intimate Sense of Smell," *National Geographic*, September 1986. Still a major landmark for the public awareness of the psychological effects of fragrances. Came with a scratch and sniff test that is still the biggest success ever of any reader's test.

D. McKenzie. *Aromatics and the Soul.* 1923.

Richard and Iona Miller. *The Magical and Ritual Use of Perfumes.* Destiny Books, Rochester, VT, 1990.

R. W. Moncrieff. *Odors.* 1970.

Edwin T. Morris. *Fragrance: The Story of Perfume from Cleopatra to Chanel.* Charles Scribner's Sons, New York, 1984.

William A. Poucher. *Perfumes, Cosmetics and Soaps*, 3 vols. Van Nostrand, Princeton, NJ, 1958.

E. Rimmel. *The Book of Perfumes.* London, 1865.

Ernest Theimer. *Fragrance Chemistry: The Science of the Sense of Smell.* Academic Press, San Diego, CA, 1982.

C. J. S. Thompson. *The Mystery and Lure of Perfumes.* J.B. Lippincott, Philadelphia, 1927.

Steve Van Toller, George Dodd. *Perfumery: The Psychology and Biology of Fragrance.* Chapman & Hall, New York, 1988. Conceived following the first international conference on the psychology of perfumery. Fascinating. The authors conduct researches at the University of Warwick in England.

Specialized Publications

Common Scents: Newsletter of the American AromaTherapy Association
P.O. Box 1222, Fair Oaks, CA 95628
Subscriptions available for nonmembers.

The International Journal of Aromatherapy
Aromatherapy Publications
3, Shirley Street
Hove, E. Sussex BN3 3WJ, England
Edited by Robert Tisserand, available through the American AromaTherapy Association.

The Journal of Essential Oil Research
Allured Publishing Corporation
P.O. Box 318, Wheaton, IL 60189-0318

Perfumer and Flavorist
Allured Publishing Corporation
P.O. Box 318, Wheaton, IL 60189-0318

Resource Guide

Associations

American AromaTherapy Association
P.O. Box 3243, South Pasadena, CA 91031
The AATA holds an annual convention, offers educational guidelines and networking for practitioners.

The Association of Tisserand Aromatherapists
44 Ditchling Rise, Brighton, E. Sussex BN1 3PY, England

International Federation of Aromatherapists
46 Dalkeith Road, Dulwich, London SE21 8LS, England

Education: Courses, Seminars, Classes, Speakers

Aromatherapy Seminar
3384 So. Robertson Place, Los Angeles, CA 90034
(800) 669-9514
Two-day beginner's seminars and 6-day advanced training.
Teachers: Marcel Lavabre, Founder, Vice President of the AATA, and Michael Scholes, professional member of the AATA.

California School of Herbal Studies
9309 HWY 116, Forestville, CA 95436
(707) 887-2012
Offers aromatherapy classes within their herbal courses.
Teachers: Jim and Mindi Green.

John Steele: Researcher, lecturer, aromatherapy consultant, custom blending, specialty oils.

Paula Dzikowski
1320 Pearl Street, Suite 120, Boulder, CO 80302
(303) 449-0191
Two-day introductory seminars and 4-day advanced training.

Esthetec
580 Lancaster Avenue, Bryn Mawr, PA 19010
(215) 525-7516
Teaches aesthetic aromatherapy.
Teacher: Kay Acuazzo, Honorary Founder of the AATA.

Fair Oaks Holistic Center & Ledet Oils
4611 Awani Court, Fair Oaks, CA 95628
(916) 965-7546
Ongoing classes on aromatherapy.
Teacher: Victoria Edwards, Founder, President of the AATA.

Pacific Institute of Aromatherapy
P.O. Box 606, San Rafael, CA 94915
(415) 459-3998
Correspondence courses, lectures, seminars.
Teacher: Kurt Schnaubelt, Ph.D., Founder, Vice President of the AATA.

Windrose
3908 E. Windrose Drive, Phoenix, AZ 85032
(602) 482-1814
Beginners and advanced training.
Teacher: Kate Damian, Honorary Founder of the AATA.
Also: Essential oils, Aromatherapy products, custom blending.

Reputable Suppliers of Essential Oils

Aroma Vera, Inc.
P.O. Box 3609, Culver City, CA 90231
(800) 669-9514
Importer of over 70 essential oils. Purchases directly from producers. Carries also the aromatic diffuser and an extensive line of aromatherapy products. Manufacturer. Bulk, wholesale, mail order, private labeling, product development.

ICB Manufacturing
311 So. Date, Alhambra, CA 91803
(818) 300-8097
Aromatherapy skin and body care, product development, private labeling. Manufacturer, wholesale.

Ledet Oils
4611 Awani Court, Fair Oaks, CA 95628
(916) 965-7546
Extensive line of essential oils and absolutes, perfume oils, massage oils. Wholesale, mail order.

Original Swiss Aromatics
Pacific Institute of Aromatherapy
P.O. Box 606, San Rafael, CA 94915
(415) 459-3998
Extensive line of essential oils, including chemotyped oils and hard-to-find oils. Wholesale, mail order.

Distributors of Quality Essential Oils

Beaute Supplies, Inc.
1421 S.W. 12th Avenue, Suite A, Pompano Beach, FL 33069
(305) 785-2680

Essential Therapeutics
37 Maud Street, P.O. Box 252
N. Balwyn, Victoria 3104, Australia
(61) 38594370

L & H Vitamins
37-10 Crescent Street, Long Island, NY 11101
(718) 937-7400
Mail order catalog.

The Preferred Source
3637 W. Alabama, Suite 160, Houston, TX 77027
(713) 622-2190

Purity Life Health Products
100 Elgin Street South, Acton, Ontario L7J 2W1, Canada
(519) 853-3511

Renaissance
2767 East Grand River, East Lansing, MI 48823
(517) 337-2023

Satau, Inc.
425 Avenue Meloche, Dorval, Quebec H9P 2W2, Canada
(514) 631-5775

True Essence Aromatherapy
1910 Bowness Road N.W., Calgary, Alberta
T2N 3K6, Canada
(403) 283-5653

Vopus Trading
Winston Churchill 295, El Senorial, Rio Piedras,
PR 00927
(809) 755-1318

Stores Carrying a Wide Variety of Quality Essential Oils

A lot has changed since this book was first published just slightly over 1 year ago. Nordstrom has now opened aromatherapy sections with a wide range of aromatherapy products in selected stores across the country. In health food stores, more and more chains are now carrying aromatherapy supplies also.

Alfalfa's Market
1651 Broadway, Boulder, CO 80302
(303) 442-0082

Alfalfa's Market
201 University Blvd., Denver, CO 80206
(303) 320-9071

Alfalfa's II
5910 S. University Blvd., Littleton, CO 80121
(303) 798-9699

Aromatherapy Scenter
33 East 20th Avenue, Eugene, OR 97405-2901
(503) 484-7058

Ayurveda Prana Foods
129 1st Avenue, New York, NY 10003
(212) 260-1218

Basic Living Products, Inc.
1321 67th Street, Emeryville, CA 94608-1120
(415) 428-1600

The Bee Hive
5807 Winfield Blvd., San Jose, CA 95123
(408) 225-3531

Bread of Life
1690 South Bascom Avenue, Campbell, CA 95008
(408) 371-5000

Capitol Drugs
4454 Van Nuys Blvd., Sherman Oaks, CA 91403
(818) 905-8338

Capitol Drugs
8578 Santa Monica Blvd., W. Hollywood, CA 90069
(213) 289-1125

Country Sun
440 California Avenue, Palo Alto, CA 94306
(415) 324-1966

Cinnabar
HWY 89–Box A, Corwin Springs, MT 59021
(406) 848-7893

Crystal Castle
313 Highway 179, Sedona, AZ 86336
(602) 282-5910

Elizabeth Luke
P.O. Box 289, Eugene, OR 97440
(503) 484-7058

Essential Images
710 Barclay Court, Ann Arbor, MI 48105
(313) 995-3113

Faith Feldman for Whisper
1020 Swarthmore Avenue, Pacific Palisades, CA 90272
(213) 454-3925

Grassroots Natural Foods
1119 Fair Oaks Avenue, South Pasadena, CA
91030
(818) 799-0512

Green Tree Grocers
3560 Mount Acadia Drive, San Diego, CA 92111
(619) 560-1975

Home Body
8500 Melrose Avenue, Los Angeles, CA 90069
(213) 659-2917

Home Body
4710 Admiralty Way, Marina Del Ray, CA 90292
(213) 823-3880

Jeffery Michael Powers Salon
206 South 5th Street, Suite 300, Ann Arbor, MI
48104
(313) 996-5585

K.M. Salon International
2911 N. Sheffield, Chicago, IL 60657
(312) 327-3429

Moment of Touch
2230 J Street, Sacramento, CA 95816
(916) 443-4011

Mother's Market
225 East 17th Street, Costa Mesa, CA 92627
(714) 631-4741

Mother's Market
19770 Beach Blvd., Huntington Beach, CA 92648
(714) 963-6667

Palmetto
1034 Montana Avenue, Santa Monica, CA 90403
(213) 395-6687

Present Moment
3546 Grand Avenue South, Minneapolis, MN
55408
(612) 824-3157

Rainbow General Store
1899 Mission Street, San Francisco, CA 94103
(415) 863-9200

Seva Market
314 E. Liberty, Ann Arbor, MI 48104
(313) 662-8686

Sonoma Mission Inn
P.O. Box 1447, Sonoma, CA 95476
(707) 938-9000

Touch the Earth
231 W. Read Street, Baltimore, MD 21201
(301) 669-1424

Wild Oats
1090 St. Francis Avenue, Santa Fe, NM 8750
(505) 983-5333

Wild Oats
2260 East Colfax, Denver, CO 80206
(303) 320-1665

Whole Foods Market
774 Emerson Street, Palo Alto, CA 94301
(415) 326-8666

Index of Essential Oils

Angelica, **113**, 33, 52, 91, 92
Aniseed, **113**, 30, 38, 52, 91, 92-93

Basil, **113**, 30, 69, 70
Bay, **113**
Benzoin, **114**
Bergamot, **114**, 27, 33, 86, 87-88, 98, 100
Birch, **114-15**, 54
Burseraceae, **54-57**, 52

Cajeput, **115**, 28, 80-81, 100
Caraway, **115**, 91, 93
Cardamom, **115**
Carrot, **115-116**, 91, 93-94
Cedarwood, **118**, 3, 52, 61, 62, 99, 100
Chamomile, **116-17**, 27, 34, 58-59, 99, 100
Cinnamon, **118**, 3, 4, 6, 30, 57, 98, 100
Cistus, **119**, 53, 57-58, 99, 100
Citronella, **119**, 26, 66
Citrus fruits, **87**, 9, 52, 98
Clary sage, **119**, 19, 27, 69, 77-78, 99, 100
Clove, **119-20**, 6, 30, 34, 80, 81, 98, 100
Compositae, **58-61**
Coniferae, **61-62**, 16, 53, 100
Coriander, **120**, 4, 28, 52, 91, 94
Cumin, **120**, 91, 94
Cypress, **120**, 19, 61, 62-63

Elemi, **121**, 54-55
Eucalyptus, **121**, 17, 26, 28, 52, 80, 81-82, 100
Everlasting, **121-22**, 58, 60

Fennel, **122**, 38, 52, 91, 94
Fir, **122-23**, 61, 63, 100
Frankincense, **123**, 3, 16, 53, 54-56, 99

Geranium, **123**, 9, 20, 28, 64-65, 99, 100
Ginger, **123-24**, 4, 65-66
Graminae, **66-68**
Grapefruit, **124**, 86, 88

Hyssop, **124**, 9, 19, 26, 28, 38, 69, 70-71

Jasmine, **124-25**, 14, 19, 52, 68-69, 99, 100
Juniper, **125**, 28, 61, 63-64

Labiatae, **69-80**, 16, 52
Lavandin, **126**, 17, 19, 69, 72
Lavender, **125-26**, 9, 14, 17, 18, 27, 28, 69, 71, 99, 100
Lemon, **126**, 33, 86, 88, 98, 100
Lemongrass, **126-27**, 20, 26, 66-67, 98
Lemon verbena. *See* Verbena
Lime, **127**, 86, 88-89, 98, 100
Litsea cubeba, **127**, 66, 67
Lovage, **127-28**, 91, 94-95

Marjoram, **128**, 14, 28, 69, 72, 99, 100
Melissa, **128-29**, 26, 69, 72-73, 100
Mints, **73-74**, 69
Mugwort, **129**, 38, 58, 60
Myrrh, **129**, 3, 4, 16, 53, 54-57, 99
Myrtaceae, **80-84**, 16, 52, 100
Myrtle, **129**, 80, 82

Neroli, **130**, 14, 19, 28, 52, 86, 87, 89, 98, 100
Niaouli, **130**, 28, 52, 80, 82-83, 100
Nutmeg, **130**, 31, 33, 80, 83, 100

Orange, **130-31**, 33, 86, 89-90, 98, 100
Oregano, **131**, 6, 69, 75

Palmarosa, **131**, 20, 28, 66, 67, 100
Patchouli, **131-32**, 69, 75-76, 99, 100
Pennyroyal, **132**, 26, 69, 73-74
Pepper, **132**, 33, 84-85
Peppermint, **132-33**, 52, 69, 73-74, 98, 100
Petitgrain, **133**, 28, 86, 90, 98, 100
Pine, **133**, 32-33, 45, 61, 64, 100

Rose, **133**, 3, 14, 17, 19, 20, 28, 52, 85-86, 100
Rosemary, **133-34**, 9, 17, 69, 76-77

Rosewood, **134**, 28, 86, 99, 100
Rutaceae, **86-90**, 16

Sage, **134-35**, 9, 17, 26, 38, 69, 78
Sandalwood, **135**, 4, 12, 35, 52, 90-91, 100
Savory, **135**
Spearmint, **135-36**, 69, 73-74
Spike (spikenard), **136**, 3, 4, 69, 71-72
Spruce, **136**, 61, 64, 100

Tangerine, **136-37**, 86, 90, 100
Tarragon, **137**, 19, 30, 58, 60-61
Tea Tree, **137**, 28, 80, 83-84
Thuja, **64**, 26, 38, 61
Thyme, **137-38**, 17, 20, 69, 78-79, 98, 100

Umbelliferae, **91-95**, 16

Verbena, **138**, 26, 95
Vetiver, **139**, 52, 66, 67-68, 99

Ylang Ylang, **139**, 14, 95-96, 99, 100

Index

Absolutes, 19, 20
Accumulation problems, 103
Acetic acid, 27
Action of aromatics, 9
Ailments, 103-111
Alchemy, 4-5
Alcohols, 17, 28
Aldehyde, 30
Aldehydes, 17, 26-27, 31
Alkaloids, 5
Allergy, 12
Allopathy, 6, 8, 9
Alpha-sabinene, 33
Alpha-terpineol, 28
Amphetamines, 5
Androsterol, 12
Anemia, 52
Anesthetic properties, 30
Anethol, 30, 31
Anosmia, 11
Anthroposophic medicine, 8, 9
  vision of plants, 48
Antibacterial properties, 35
Antibiotic properties, 6
Antibiotics, 2, 5, 17
Anticarcinogenic properties, 9, 30, 34
Antidepressants, 5

Antifungal properties, 27
Antigenetic properties, 7
Antineuralgic properties, 9
Antiphlogistic properties, 34
Antiseptic properties, 4, 6, 7, 9, 26, 28, 30, 32, 34, 45
Antiseptics, 2, 3, 17
Antiviral properties, 28, 33, 34
Anxiety, 14, 108
Aphrodisiac, 9
Apiol, 30, 31
Apocrine glands, 11-12
Armond, A. D., 13-14
Aromasols, 43
Aromatogram, 6-7
Articular problems, 104
Asteraceae family, 34
Astral body, 9, 52, 99
  formulas for, 111
Avicenna (philosopher), 4, 17
Ayurvedic medicine, 4

Bacteriostatic properties, 34
Balsamic, 3
Bath oils, 17, 41
Baths, 40-41
Bile, 9
Bisabolol, 33-34

Blending of essential oils, 97-102
   and preparations for use, 100-102
   in therapy, 14
Blood circulation, 38, 43, 106
Body
   effects of chemicals on, 8
   effects of essential oils on, 9
   internal equillibrium, 8
Body wrap, 43
Bonding of electrons, 24
Borneol, 20, 28
Bornyl acetate, 27
Botanical families, 48, 50-52
   and production of essential oils, 51-52
Brain
   and olfaction, 10-11
   treatment of diseases of, 38
Brain stimulation, 108

Calming properties, 9, 14, 27
Camphene, 32
Camphor, 31
Carbon, 23-24, 25
Carbon dioxide. *See* hypercritical carbon dioxide
   extraction
Carboxyl group, 26, 27
Carnation, 19
Carotol, 33
Carriers, 100-102
Carvacrol, 20, 28
Carvone, 26
Caryophyllen, 30, 33-34
Cassia, 19
Castoreum, 12
Cell regeneration, 41
Central nervous system, 31
Ceremonial use of aromatics, 3-5, 13, 44-45, 53
Chakras, 99
   formulas for, 111
Chamazulen, 33
Chemistry of essential oils, 7, 17, 24-34
Chemotherapy, 8
Cineol, 20, 28, 31
Cinnamic, 30

Circulatory system, 38, 45
Citral, 20, 26
Citronellal, 26
Citronellol, 28
Citrus oils, 32
Civet, 12
Cohobation, 21
Cold pressure extraction, 17, 21
Concretes, 19, 20
Corticosteroids, 5
Cosmetics, 9, 19, 38, 53
   history of, 3, 5
   use of essential oils in, 20-21, 41-44
Creativity, 13

Deep relaxation, 14
Deodorizing properties, 34
Depression, 11, 14
   formulas for, 108
Dermatophilic properties, 34
Diagnosis, 15
Diffusion of essential oils, 14, 44-45
Digestive system, 11, 38, 52, 106
Dilution, 19, 38-39
Dioscorides, 17-18
Disinfection, 21
Distillates, 21
Distillation, 20
   and chemistry of essential oils, 25
   of flowers, 52
   history, 4-5, 17-18
   methods, 18, 21-22
   quality of yield, 21
Diterpenes, 25-26, 33
Dodd, G. H., 6, 12
Dosage, 38-39
Double filtration, 19
Douek, E., 11

Egyptian use of aromatics, 3-4, 17
Elimination problems, 103
Embalming, 4
Emotional behavior, 11
   formulas for, 108

Endocrine glands, 8
Energizing properties, 28
Energy formulas, 109, 111
Enfleurage, 17
Equilibrating qualities, 52
Equisetaceae, 48
Essential oils, 1, 6, 7, 14, 16, 20-21
  antiseptic properties of, 6-7
  blending of, 97-100
  ceremonial use of, 3-5, 13, 44-45, 53
  chemistry of, 7, 17, 24-34
  classification of, 7, 25-34, 49, 98
  effect on body of, 9
  extraction of, 17-22
  history of, 3-5, 40-41
  in plants, 8-9, 51-52
  preparations for use, 100-102
  qualities of, 52-53
  storage of, 22, 103
  therapeutic use of, 13-14, 15
  use of, 38-47
Esters, 17, 27, 31
Estragol, 28
Estrogen, 9
Estrone, 9
Ethyl alcohol, 38-39
Eucalyptole, 28
Eugenol, 28, 30
External use of essential oils, 39-41
Extraction of essential oils, 17-22
  see also distillation

Facial care, 43
Farnesol, 33-34
Feminine cycle, 104
Fixatives, 99
Floral production of essential oils, 52
Floral waters, 21, 42, 43
Food industry, 20-21
Formulas for ailments, 103-111
Fragrances, 13, 15
  plant production of, 52
Freud, Sigmund, 12
Functional groups, 26-37
Fungicidal properties, 30

Gaia hypothesis, 50, 51
Gamma-terpinene, 33
Garlic, 9
Gattefosse, R.M., 5, 6
Genetic theory, 8
Geranial, 26
Geraniol, 20, 28
Geranyl acetate, 27
Ginseng, 9
Girault, Maurice, 5, 6-7, 15
Glandular system, 53
Gums, 53
Gynecology, 7

Hair care, 38, 44
  formulas for, 110
Hallucinogen, 31
Headaches, 106
Healing properties, 17, 21, 53
Heart, 38
Herbal energy, 1
Herbal therapy, 5
Herpes simplex, 32
Hexane, 19
Hippocrates, 8, 45
Homeopathy, 8, 15, 48
Homeostasis, 8
Honeysuckle, 19
Hops, 9
Hormones, 8, 17
  in essential oils, 9
Hydrogen, 23
Hydrolates, 21
Hydroxyl group, 28
Hypercritical carbon dioxide extraction, 19-20
Hypnosis, 14
Hypnotics, 5
Hypothalamic region, 12

Impotence, 106
Indian use of aromatics, 4
Infectious diseases, 7, 38, 106
Ingestion, 38
Inhalation, 44-45
Injection, 38

Insect repellents, 107
Internal use of essential oils, 38-39
Intoxicating qualities, 52
Invigorating qualities, 45, 52
Isoprene, 25

Kephi, 3
Ketones, 17, 26, 31

Labdanum, 3
Lauraceae, 16
Leaf production of essential oils, 52
Lemery, Nicholas, 5
Licorice, 9
Limbic system, 10-11
Limonene, 32
Linalol, 20, 27, 28
Linalyl acetate, 27
Lungs, 38

Massage, 3, 14, 27
   use of essential oils in, 38, 39-40
Massage oils, 17, 39-40
Mastick, 33
Maury, Marguerite, 9, 41
Medicine, 4, 5, 7, 8
Meditation, 14, 53
   formulas for, 111
Memory
   and Gaia hypothesis, 51
   and olfaction, 13
Memory of molecules, 49
Menstruation, 9, 12
   formulas for, 104
Methylchavicol, 30, 31
Methyl salicilate, 27
Microorganisms, 7, 34
Mind and aromatics, 9
Monoterpenes, 25-26, 28-30, 33
Morphogenetic fields, 49-50
Mucus flow, 26
Muscular problems, 104
Musk, 12

Myrcene, 32
Myristicin, 30, 31

Narcissus, 52
Nebulizer, 38
Neral, 26
Nerol, 28
Nerolidol, 20
Nutrition, 15

Oil. *See* bath oils; essential oils; massage oils
Oleoresins, 20
Olfaction, 10-12
   anatomy of, 10
   and diagnosis, 15
   and psychotherapy, 13-14
   and sexuality, 11-12, 12
   and the unconcious, 12-13
Organic zcids, 17
Oxidation, 32, 45
Oxides, 28
Oxygen, 23

Paraclesus, 8, 48
Paranoia, 11
Parosmia, 11
Parsley, 9, 31
Perfumery, 9, 12, 19
   history of, 4, 5
   use of oils in, 21
Pesticides, 21
Phenols, 17, 28-30, 31
Phenylpropane derivatives, 25, 30-31
Pheromones, 11-12, 12
Phoenicians, 3
Pinene, 33
Pinocamphone, 26
Plants, 2, 8, 14, 21, 51
   biochemistry of, 9, 20
   classification of, 48
   effects of essential oils on, 16
   productions of essential oils in, 51-52
   therapeutic properites of, 8

Prajna energy, 52
Pressure cooker, 21
Principle of opposites, 8
Principle of similarities, 8
Production of essential oils, 51-53
Psychoanalysis, 12
Psychoaromatherapy, 14
Psychology of smell, 11
Psychotherapy, 13-14, 15
Pulegone, 26

Qualities of essential oils, 52-53
Quality of essential oils, 20-21

Rancidity, 103
Reconstituted oil, 20-21
Refrigerated coil, 4, 18
Religious use of aromatics, 3-5, 13, 44-45, 53
Resins, 53
Resistance phenomena, 7
Respiratory system, 26, 38, 45, 52
    treatments for, 105
Root production of essential oils, 52
Rosaceae, 48
Rousseau, Jean-Jacques, 13
Rue, 38

Safrol, 30, 31
St. John's Wort, 17
Salvia, 77
Santalol, 28, 33, 35
Sassafras, 31
Science and herbal therapy, 5, 6
Sedative properties, 26, 27, 34
Seed production of essential oils, 52
Sesquiterpenes, 17, 25-26, 33-35
Sexuality and olfaction, 11-12
Shyness, 11
Skin absorbtion, 39-40
Skin care, 21, 26, 34, 38, 53
    formulas for use, 42-43, 110
    history of, 3, 5
    use of essential oils in, 41-44

Skin irritation, 30, 32, 41
Smell. *See* olfaction
Solvent extraction, 19, 20, 21, 52
Soul amd aromatics, 9
Spasmolytic properties, 27
Steam distillation. *See* distillation
Stearine, 20
Steiner, Rudolf, 8
    See also anthroposophic medicine
Stimulant properties, 9
Stoddart, D. M., 12
Storage of essential oils, 22, 103
Stress, 14, 108
Synergy, 97-98
Synthetic antibiotics, 7
Synthetic oils, 20-21, 49
    and effect on body, 7

Tehuti (Egyptian god), 4
Temperature, 22
Terpene alcohols, 20, 28, 31
Terpene hydrocarbons, 32
Terpenes, 17, 25
Terpenoid, 30, 31
Terpineol-4, 28
Thujone, 26
Thymol, 20, 28
Tisserand, Robert, 14, 41
Toxicity, 26, 28, 31, 52
Tranquilizer, 3
Treatment of organs, 38
Tree bark production of essential oils, 52-53
Tuberose, 19, 52
Turpentine, 33

Ulcers, 53
Unconcious and olfaction, 12-13
Urinary tract, 34

Valnet, Jean, 5, 7, 9
Vedas, 4
Virel, Andre, 13

Viruses, 32
Vitamins, 17

Waxes, 19
Wintergreen, 54
Wood production of essential oils, 52-53
Wounds, 53

Yoga, 14, 53, 111

Zingiberol, 33
Zozime (Egyptian chemist), 17

THE ART OF AROMATHERAPY

The Healing and Beautifying Properties of the Essential Oils of Flowers and Herbs
Robert B. Tisserand

"Standard reference work since it was published..." —**Vogue**

Bestselling author Robert Tisserand unlocks the hidden strength of flowers and herbs in this complete guidebook, reviving the ancient and nearly forgotten art of healing with essential oils. Learn how to create massage oils, medicinal compounds, ointments, skin treatments, and aromatic baths to treat more than one hundred conditions in a safe, gentle, and effective way.

ISBN 0-89281-001-7
$10.95 paperback

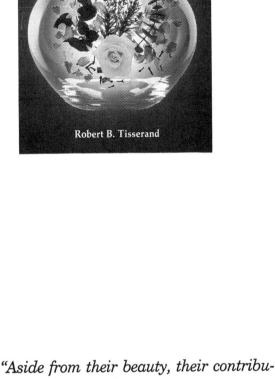

THE PRACTICE OF AROMATHERAPY

A Classic Compendium of Plant Medicines and Their Healing Properties
Jean Valnet, M.D.
Edited by Robert Tisserand

One of the world's acknowledged experts in plant medicine, Dr. Valnet details more than forty plants and essences useful in the treatment of illness and the relief of pain, including their history, properties, uses, and methods of application. With more than thirty years of work with plant essences, he shows how this ancient therapy can be an effective adjunct to modern medicine.

ISBN 0-89281-398-9
$10.95 paperback

"Aside from their beauty, their contributions to poetry and romance, flowers and herbs have long been noted for their healing properties. Discover the wonders of floral remedies and some very unconventional, but often effective, medicine."

–**Harper's Bazaar**

AROMATHERAPY FOR WOMEN

A Practical Guide to Essential Oils for Health and Beauty
Maggie Tisserand

"A very attractive handbook which will lead you into the sensual delights of essential oils and their usefulness." –**Health World**

This easy-to-use guide offers an introduction to the many uses of aromatherapy at home, with an emphasis on remedies for women and children. Here is a wealth of simple preparations to enhance sensuality, improve appearance, and alleviate health problems.

ISBN 0-89281-244-3
$6.95 paperback

AROMATHERAPY HANDBOOK

For Beauty, Hair, and Skin Care
Erich Keller

Prepare your own natural and health-giving cosmetics and personal care products with the information presented in this complete guide. The author explains the healing properties of essential oils and gives recipes for creating your own favorite combinations.

ISBN 0-89281-433-0
$12.95 paperback

These and other Inner Traditions/Healing Arts Press titles are available at many fine bookstores or, to order direct, send a check or money order for the total amount, plus $2.00 shipping and handling for the first book and $1.00 for each additional book, to:

Inner Traditions/Healing Arts Press
One Park Street
Rochester, VT 05767

A complete catalog of books is available on request.
